Keep It Simple, Keep It Whole
Your Guide to Optimum Health

Published by Exsalus Health & Wellness Center

Cover design by Monica Richards

ISBN: 978-0-615-33046-4

First edition: October 2009
Revised edition: June 2010
Printed in the United States of America

Authors' note:
The information presented in this book is for educational purposes only. It should not be considered as specific medical, nutritional, lifestyle, or other health-related advice for anyone and is not given as such. You should make medical, nutritional, lifestyle, or other health-related changes only under the care of your personal physician.

This book is dedicated to

Robi Pulde
(1949-2004)

my beloved father and my continued inspiration

ത

Acknowledgements:

To Gil Pulde, Mona Howard, and Cathy Fisher for the many hours spent transforming this book into a version we are proud to put our names on.

To John McDougall, MD, thank you for all of your guidance, support, and tutelage, without which we would not be where we are today.

We are forever indebted to you.

About the Authors

Drs. Alona Pulde and Matthew Lederman are licensed medical physicians practicing nutrition and lifestyle medicine in Los Angeles, California. Their clinic, Exsalus Health & Wellness Center, empowers patients to achieve and maintain their optimum health—physically, emotionally, and medically—through a comprehensive, patient-centered approach.

Alona and Matt are passionate promoters of nutrition and lifestyle medicine. This husband and wife team has participated in many projects, including lecturing for the eCornell Certificate Program in Plant Based Nutrition, treating patients followed in the films *Healing Cancer* and *Forks over Knives*, and answering nutrition and health questions for popular websites. Currently, they are collaborating with T. Colin Campbell on their next book, a follow-up to *The China Study*, addressing common and prevalent nutrition and lifestyle questions. In addition, they are the first doctors to ever work with John McDougall, MD, seeing patients during his 10-day live-in programs. Dr. Lederman also sits on the board of directors for the American College of Lifestyle Medicine.

Whether their medical practice is being spotlighted by a prominent lifestyle medicine organization or they are being touted as the medical practice of the future, it is clear that Drs. Pulde and Lederman are true patient advocates.

Table of Contents

Preface

Dr. Pulde's story...

For as long as I can remember I have wanted to be a doctor. Maybe that had something to do with the doctor's kit my parents gave me for my fourth birthday. It took no time at all for that toy to become my favorite pastime, as witnessed by the line of teddy bears and dolls waiting to see Dr. Alona. At the time, I obviously knew nothing about medicine, but the ability to help and heal others resonated with me.

Time elapsed and I grew into and out of many things, but one thing remained constant: my desire and my determination to help and heal people in need. So I went to UCLA to complete my undergraduate pre-med training. It was here that I received my first slap in the face as I realized that medicine had become a business more interested in making money by selling pills and procedures than caring for and advocating for patients' rights and well-being. The doctor-patient relationship depicted best in the paintings of Norman Rockwell had disintegrated as doctors were relegated to 10-15 minutes per patient and patients were restricted to just one complaint. It was no wonder these quick-fix methods were not producing successes and that patients were delving deeper into their chronic illnesses, relying more and more on medications and "life-saving" procedures. I was devastated, as this was *not* the medicine I had so anticipated practicing.

Fortunately, at the same time that I was coming to this disappointing realization, I happened to be volunteering at a shelter for patients with HIV and AIDS. There, I was working with an acupuncturist who was teaching me a completely different approach to medicine. She not only spent an hour with each patient, focusing on their needs, concerns, and ailments, but she treated them in a comprehensive manner that addressed their physical, mental, and emotional well-being. And her results were astonishing! No, she didn't cure them of their disease, but she did alleviate a lot of the suffering associated with their illness as well as the side effects caused by their medications. Equally important, her patients felt heard, taken care of,

1

and supported. THIS was the medicine I had always envisioned practicing, and so I pursued an education in Chinese Medicine.

The four years that I spent at Emperor's College getting my degree in Traditional Chinese Medicine, including acupuncture and herbology, were some of the best years I have ever spent. For the first time in my adult life I was doing something I absolutely loved and completely believed in. Life was almost perfect. Why almost? Because throughout my training, my greatest mentor, Dr. Xiuling Ma, believed that the only way to truly provide comprehensive medical care to patients was to combine Eastern and Western medicines. That was how she learned and what made her so competent in her practice. And so, after some deliberation, I went back to school to get my medical degree.

Medical school proved to be one of the best and one of the worst experiences in my life. Best because Dr. Ma was absolutely correct that in order to be a comprehensive healthcare provider it is helpful to know, understand, and practice both Eastern and Western medicines. The knowledge and the experience that I attained while in medical school are invaluable to my practice today—invaluable but, unfortunately, incomplete.

My second slap in the face came after finishing my second year of medical school. This time it was a much more personal devastation; the sudden death of my beloved father. With all my training and all my knowledge I could not understand for the life of me how a healthy man like my dad could suddenly die of a heart attack at age 55. Yes, he had high cholesterol, but it was managed with cholesterol-lowering medication, and other than that, he was in terrific health. After all, we lived in a home that followed (for the most part) the Mediterranean diet. We ate tons of fruits, vegetables, and olive oil. We exercised regularly. We followed the recommended guidelines, hoping to reduce our cholesterol and fat intakes even more by eating chicken, turkey, and fish instead of beef and lamb; and our dairy intake was limited to occasional cheeses and ice cream. So, how could this happen? I was consumed with rage—what was this medicine (philosophy, pharmacology, and practice) worth if it couldn't allow a seemingly healthy and beloved husband, father, and friend to live to a ripe old age? Obviously, I was missing something; but what could it be?

Again, as luck, or maybe this time fate (thanks Dad!), would have it, I met Matt (my incredible husband). I was fortunate to have crossed his path, for more reasons than one, as he happened to have the answers I was looking for. Through his wisdom and his passion I was introduced to the works of John McDougall, MD, T. Colin Campbell, PhD, and Caldwell Esselstyn, MD, among others. Suddenly, I was awakened to a world were medicine was again making a difference in people's lives. Patients were not only losing weight but were getting rid of their medications as they *reversed* their heart disease and cancer, *cured* their diabetes, and *reduced* their blood pressure and cholesterol. How were they doing this? Through diet and lifestyle changes—specifically, by adopting a low-fat, whole foods, plant-based diet while eliminating animal products, oils, refined and processed foods, and bad habits (like smoking). The more I read the more I was enthralled, because for every argument I had (Where will I get my protein? Isn't olive oil good for you? What about calcium? But, aren't chicken and fish healthy?), these doctors had an answer and the evidence to prove it. I evaluated the evidence only to find that they were right *every* time, although I really only needed to look at the success they were having with their patients to know what they were saying was true.

So, thanks to Matt and the doctors he so revered, my passion for medicine was reawakened. Finally, I had discovered the path that would allow me to be the doctor I had always wanted to be—one who can truly help patients by giving them the tools to heal themselves.

As with many things in life, this was a bittersweet realization. Bitter, in that I wish I had known this information sooner, as it may have saved the life of my beloved father. But sweet because I now have the opportunity to share this knowledge with the rest of my family and my friends, and you and your loved ones in hopes that it will help you live the long, healthy, and happy life you deserve.

Dr. Lederman's story...

I had never really considered any other profession, as I had always thought I was going to be a cardiologist, just like my father. Helping sick patients, participating in life-changing research, and being an educated resource to those in need drew me into this challenging profession. Unfortunately, after four years of medical school and four years of practicing medicine, I grew disillusioned and was ready to leave medicine altogether. I do not know what was to blame, be it the frustrations that come with a practice so driven by the pharmaceutical industry and the insurance industry or the simple fact that patients were not getting better despite delivering the best care available. The medicine that I was practicing had very little to do with my original motivations to become a doctor.

Additionally, I felt lousy. I was physically ill. I couldn't go through a day without feeling awful. My stomach was my worst enemy. I was given the vague diagnosis of Irritable Bowel Syndrome, taking pill after pill to reduce the stubborn symptoms. Nothing worked. My diet was healthy according to modern medicine. I even removed lactose as much as possible, except when my cravings kicked in. My diet "hiccup" was a double barbeque bacon cheeseburger and fries followed by ice cream. Every once in a while wouldn't hurt, I thought; those foods were treats!

I had already experienced my fair share of medical procedures and blood tests, looking for other potential causes of my escalating symptoms. I even went to integrative physicians trying all sorts of alternative medications. I was considering yet another invasive procedure when my father reminded me of the risks involved. I was desperate, under the impression that more procedures would ultimately provide an answer. However, he challenged me to at least experiment with eliminating alcohol and junk foods before proceeding. He wasn't sure what diet to recommend but was sure that more medical care was clearly not the answer. Moreover, from a cardiologist's point of view, it couldn't hurt to at least stop the alcohol and fast food.

I committed *only* to doing some research. I went to the bookstore and read about nutrition and health, a topic overlooked in most medical schools. I was fascinated by the claims made by so many medical nutrition experts: reverse chronic disease, lose weight without dieting, lower cholesterol without medication, etc. "Craziness," I thought, "likely just a bunch of medical quacks trying to sell an easy answer."

Thankfully, I was stubborn and determined to prove the medical nutrition experts wrong. I continued my research and exploration of medical journals and studies. I discovered that these experts told the truth, which was a hard truth for me to digest. I contacted Dr. John McDougall, one of the leading medical nutrition experts in the country, who has a successful practice in Northern California promoting plant-based nutrition as a medical strategy. Dr. McDougall kindly invited me to observe his practice and I accepted.

I thank Dr. McDougall for reigniting my passion in medicine. His practice embodied my childhood understanding of what medicine should look and feel like. His patients were engaged in the process of becoming healthy and were empowered to make lifestyle changes. His patients were happy, excited, and thoroughly supported. As a result of following the McDougall program, his patients were reversing chronic diseases, losing weight, and seeing significantly improved blood test results. In my new excitement and enthusiasm, I decided that nutrition-based lifestyle medicine was the only way I could continue practicing medicine.

Somewhere in the process, I discovered that my stomach symptoms undeniably correlated to my diet. Animal products (dairy, eggs, meat), processed foods, and oil triggered painful reactions. Plant-based, whole foods were a joy to eat in comparison. It was an easy decision to hold off on further medical procedures, opting instead to continue with my nutrition experiment.

I committed to eating a plant-based, whole foods diet. Unfortunately, these foods were hard to come by, even in health-conscious Los Angeles. Most vegan restaurants doused their food in oils and depended highly on processed foods (meat substitutes galore). Additionally, despite my abilities to perform complex medical procedures, I could barely turn on my stove. At first I ate simple plant-based whole foods: oats, rice, beans, fruits, and vegetables. I ate what I could cook. But after about a week, my willpower ran out. I was miserably deprived. In a moment of frustration, after passing my favorite fast food drive-in, I succumbed to a double barbeque bacon cheeseburger and fries. The resulting pain reminded me that this food was far from harmless.

I committed to trying plant-based whole foods again, only this time I needed to arm myself with the tools to succeed. If eating out was not a regular option, I needed to learn how to cook. I started slowly and learned to cook one recipe at a time. I learned how to be forgiving, as there were some meals I wouldn't wish upon my worst enemy. Each "failure" was a new lesson. Each lesson helped me reach my ultimate goal of feeling healthy and happy. Failure was just not an option.

Without even trying, I lost weight. At 6 feet tall I weighed 195 pounds when I started my new diet and lifestyle, and am now a lean 180 pounds. My stomach troubles are also under control, so long as I follow a diet filled with whole foods. My blood test results are impressive. But, more so, I am happy. I enjoy what I eat, and I love that I am pain-free and finally have some control over my health.

Despite my success, I received a lot of criticism and judgment from my medical colleagues, my peers, and even my family. It's been a hard journey. I am aware of how crazy my claims may sound to newcomers. But, trust me; I'm a doctor. Actually (in all seriousness), never trust anyone who tells you to trust them simply because they are a doctor. Trust how you feel, the results you see, the happiness you derive, and hopefully, unbiased science. I've studied and researched what most doctors don't ever think about: the relationship between nutrition and food and the human body. Armed with facts, research, and healthy recipes I've helped my family, friends, and colleagues understand how to transition to health.

I truly believe that things happen for a reason. I believe that I was meant to be a doctor. I also believe that my Irritable Bowel Syndrome was a signal that I was damaging my body with an unhealthy, disease-promoting lifestyle. Though awful, my stomach pain was the catalyst to my becoming both a healthier person and a better physician. Most importantly, I believe that I met Alona, my beautiful wife, for a reason. It is hard to argue that things don't happen for a reason, as we were clearly meant to be together, both from a personal and professional standpoint. We have continued our journey together hand in hand as we opened our first clinic, Exsalus Health & Wellness Center in Los Angeles, California. We share a similar vision of opening health & wellness centers around the world that focus on treating patients utilizing the Exsalus Health Program.

Alona and I are physicians with no ulterior motives. We are focused on being true patient advocates. We are not selling anything other than solid, researched facts; the decision of what to do with those facts is up to our patients, not us. We provide the road map that directs our patients where they want and need to go, and then support them along the way as they achieve their optimum health. Ultimately, we refuse to offer anything other than the safest, most effective, and evidence-based medicine available.

In this book you are about to read, Alona has done a fantastic job summarizing the information we have assembled over the years into a fun and easy guide of the basics you will need to get started. Take this foundation of new information and add to it what you learn during your own personal journey. Our goal here is to provide enough information to allow you to feel comfortable with the decision to make these health changes without being so overwhelmed that you never get started. I only wish I had this easy-to-use resource when I was in your shoes. So please enjoy, and get excited to look and feel the way you always wanted as you begin your path to achieving optimum health.

Introduction

Thank you for opening this book and congratulations. Congratulations because you have just embarked on a journey to recapture your health. To quote one of our patients, this journey is "nothing short of incredible." In the following chapters, you will find answers to many of your greatest medical and health concerns. You will learn how to reverse heart disease, cancer, diabetes, and high blood pressure, among other illnesses. You will learn how to slim down to your natural trim weight without diets, starvation, or deprivation. You will learn how to overcome fatigue to finally have the energy you desire. You will learn how the medical/pharmaceutical industry deceives you and how buying into their business can leave you sick or sicker than you were to begin with. And empowered with this new information, you will have the tools you need to become the healthy person you have always hoped to be.

The information in this book may be news to many, if not most of you. As such, while you read this book, we have only one request:

> "To scrutinize what we say is requested but to condemn it without investigation is folly."[1]

In fact, we encourage you to question, challenge, and investigate our claims, and we are confident that in doing so, you will reach our same conclusions. That being said, let's get started. Ladies and gentlemen,

the state of our health is going from bad to worse.

For the first time in history, parents are outliving their children.[2] Americans are spending more money on healthcare yet are getting fatter and sicker.[3] Two-thirds of adults are currently overweight, and of those, half are obese.[4] In fact, it is estimated that if we continue at this rate, ALL Americans will be overweight by 2050 and ALL Americans will be obese by the end of the century.[5] That even extends to our children, since over the last 30 years childhood obesity has tripled, and children are heavier than they have ever been.[6] As if this isn't bad enough, regardless of the money being pumped into medical research and technological advancement, our biggest health killers remain Heart Disease (#1) and Cancer (#2).

What does this tell us? It tells us that,

whatever we've been doing until now
is NOT working and, more importantly,
we need to try something new.

So, why don't we? What keeps us in the same old rut? For some of us, it is lack of knowledge: we don't realize we need to change. For others, it is lack of motivation: we know what we should do and why but can't muster up the energy to get going. But for most of us, it is our ambiguity, a perpetual state of confusion in which we know we need to change but we are not sure how or how well it will work for us. And this is completely understandable in light of the fact that every day we are bombarded with messages from the media, celebrities, family, and friends. Today protein is in and carbs are out, while yesterday it was the exact opposite. So, what do we do? Do we clean out the kitchen once more to accommodate this new "fad" or do we wait for tomorrow; maybe protein will be back and we can keep our turkey sausages and chicken wings. The uncertainty alone could drive us crazy enough to maintain our routine without making ANY changes. But that, my friends, is definitely not the solution.

You wouldn't be reading this book if you were looking to stay in status quo. No, you are looking to make changes, real, permanent, healthy changes, not the quick-fix "today you are in and tomorrow you're out" kind of changes. And that is where we step in, because we at Exsalus Health & Wellness Center can help you find your solution. So, hop in, buckle your seatbelts, and get ready for the ride of your life! Before we begin, here are a few tips to help you navigate through this book:

1) It is extremely important to us that our information is evidence-based. As such, we include and discuss many studies in this book. We feel this is an integral part of the learning process. It is one thing for us to tell you what to do (and for you to take our word for it) and a completely different thing for you to really understand why you are doing it. An analogy would be imagining a child eating dirt. When they are young, we tell them not to do so and they must take our word for it, versus when they are older and able to understand why they should not be eating dirt, and they make that informed decision for themselves. Although the former works, the latter is much

more effective at achieving long-term compliance. Having said that, we recognize that reviewing medical research is not for everyone. So, for those of you that are interested in the research, this will be a great opportunity to become familiar with the literature. And, for those of you more interested in the bottom line, feel free to skim or skip over the studies. Regardless of the approach you choose, the take-home message remains the same.

2) In writing this book, we hope to reach as wide an audience as possible, as we truly believe everyone can benefit from learning the information provided throughout these pages. However, in doing so, we recognize that we are appealing to a broad spectrum of people with different interests, personalities, and time constraints. Some of you will be global processors interested in the big picture, others will be detail-oriented and will focus in on the specifics, and still others will just want to get to the bottom line. Because we feel it is important, we spent a significant amount of time answering the question, "Why do we need this information?" before actually introducing the Exsalus Health Program. This is because we believe that it is so much more empowering for you to know why you are doing something versus just taking our word for it. So, for those of you interested in the "why?" you will want to read the book in order from Chapter 1 to Chapter 14. But, for those of you just interested in the "how" or the crux of the program, you may want to begin reading from Chapter 7 and, if interested, at a later date return to the beginning chapters (this will be helpful if you find down the road that you are struggling with staying on the program).

3) Our goal in writing this book is to share the information we have learned over the years and believe to be the best path to optimum health. For many of you, this information represents a radical alternative to your current diet and lifestyle. As such, you may find it overwhelming at first and become discouraged. But, keep in mind as you read that learning this new diet and lifestyle is like learning a new language. You don't become fluent in a new language overnight. On the contrary, it takes time and even more than time, it takes practice. Furthermore, while you are learning and practicing a new language, you are bound to make mistakes. This will apply to the Exsalus Health Program as well. In the same way that it would take time to perfect your accent, it will take time to learn to make delicious and healthy meals. And in the same way that mispronouncing a word doesn't mean the language is impossible to learn, ruining

or making a bad dish doesn't mean this diet doesn't work or cannot be tasty. We, and the many people whose lives have already been changed by this program (see Testimonials in Appendix J), would not be living this way if we weren't reaping the many rewards of this healthy and delicious new diet and lifestyle. So, keep in mind that this will be a work in progress, but also know that by reading and applying the recommendations in this book you **can**, and you **will**, become fluent in this new language of optimum health.

Note: The information presented in this book is for educational purposes only. It should not be considered as specific medical, nutritional, lifestyle, or other health-related advice for anyone and is not given as such. You should make medical, nutritional, lifestyle, or other health-related changes ONLY under the care of your personal physician.

Chapter 1: It Starts with Nutrition

The honest truth is: It starts with nutrition. We, like cars and other such machines, run on fuel. For us, that fuel is food and water. It is easy enough for us to know our car needs gasoline and not dishwasher soap. So, why is it so difficult for us to understand that we need nutritious whole foods and not cheeseburgers, sodas, and donuts? The reality is that this is not our fault. Our bodies are not flawed. This is not a problem resulting from defective genes, inability to portion control, or a propensity to emotionally eat. Instead,

the problem lies in the environment we currently live in.

You see, we are inherently hard-wired to enjoy pleasurable experiences, which served as a very useful survival mechanism for our ancestors. We will elaborate on this soon, but to summarize the idea, in order for our ancestors to survive in nature, they needed to learn how to find food without becoming food. The most efficient way to do this was to find the foods with the most calories. For example, if they had a choice between a banana and a cucumber, they were programmed to choose the banana. Why was this such a useful survival tool? Because, we only need a certain amount of calories a day, let's say 2000 calories. That would mean either about 20 bananas or about 45 cucumbers. By going for the banana, our ancestors would get the most bang for their buck; they would have to work less to get the right amount of food, and by saving time, they would limit their exposure to outdoor danger. So, the banana became a win-win choice. Unfortunately, the advancements in our environment have created new scenarios for us. We are no longer choosing between a banana and a cucumber; instead, we are choosing between a banana and a cheeseburger. And, using the same algorithm, it now becomes more understandable why we choose the cheeseburger.

Okay, so now we understand why we make certain food choices, but what does this have to do with experiencing pleasure beyond that of food tasting good, and how does it actually harm us?

> When we experience pleasure, a neurotransmitter
> called dopamine is released in our brain.[7]

This happens with any pleasurable experience, from falling in love to being intimate to winning the lottery to eating an ice cream sundae. The release of dopamine is what we then interpret as pleasure and what propels us into a dopamine-pleasure cycle.[8]

> During the dopamine-pleasure cycle
> we release dopamine, we feel good, we continue
> doing the action that will release dopamine,
> and we continue to feel pleasure.

Through pleasure reinforcement, this mechanism ensures that we continue to repeat those behaviors that are necessary for our survival; for example eating and reproducing. But, those are not the only activities that release dopamine in our brain. In fact, over time

> we have learned how to manipulate this system
> with cocaine, heroin and, unknowingly, with
> our favorite fast food version of a heart attack on a plate.

So, we can begin to see that a system that may have worked for our ancestors (who didn't have fast food restaurants and drug dealers so readily available) may not work so well for us.

Let's explore this a little more. We want to feel good; who wouldn't? In fact, up until the last 100 years or so, whatever made us feel good was generally in our evolutionary best interest. So, as we discussed above, it is in our nature to turn to those things that will give us pleasure, one of which is the food we eat. The problem is that the more calorie-dense the food (has more calories per square inch), the more dopamine is released.

Figure 1 - The Caloric Density of Various Foods (how many calories per 100 grams of a given food)

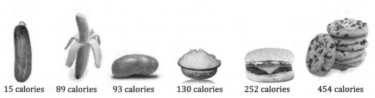

15 calories   89 calories   93 calories   130 calories   252 calories   454 calories

Again, this works well for ensuring our survival. Given a choice of a cucumber or a banana, our ancestors were encouraged to choose the banana. But this was because, as we mentioned earlier, for them, it was dangerous (possibly life-threatening) to go out and get food. In addition, food was not as readily available, and storing extra calories for "rainy days" was a reality and often a necessity for survival. In today's world, with no saber tooth tiger lurking in the shadows and with fast food restaurants and convenience stores at every corner, we no longer share those concerns. But, our body is still programmed to seek out caloric density. What our body doesn't realize is that we are no longer only choosing from whole foods; rather, many of us rely on fast foods or processed/packaged foods for breakfast, lunch, and dinner or some combination thereof.

We are programmed to seek caloric density, BUT we are no longer choosing from whole foods.

So, why is that a problem, you may ask? Well, let's put aside the abundance of cholesterol and fat in these foods, two primary constituents for developing heart disease. Let's table the loads of sugar and salt poured into these foods that contribute to problems like high blood pressure and diabetes. And let's even shelve, for now, the environmental contaminants found in these foods (from E. coli to dioxin) that can cause anything from stomach upset to cancer and death. What we are focusing on here is just calorie density.

Our stomach responds to two things: stretch and calories.

Based on this information, we have a built-in system that assesses how many calories we need in a given day.

This system is very accurate as long as we are eating **natural whole foods**,

our "calorie currency" per se. But, when we introduce fast food and junk food into our bodies, our system goes haywire. This is primarily because when manufacturers process food, they remove water and fiber along with other nutrients, which condenses calories so that the stretch of the stomach and calorie density no longer correlate. If you eat 500 calories of potatoes (see Figure 2) your stomach will be stretched significantly, and as a result you will feel full.

However, if you eat 500 calories of beef or 500 calories of chocolate, both devoid of fiber and water (see Figure 2), they do not fill up your stomach and you will continue to feel hungry. Your body will be confused (by the lack of stretch) into believing it has not consumed enough calories, and it will instruct you to eat more. You cannot fight this survival instinct, just as you cannot breathe five times per minute for an extended period of time if your brain says you need ten breaths per minute. So, you eat to not feel hungry, but by the end of the meal you have consumed more calories than your body actually needed. Over time, this results in weight gain.

3500 additional calories equals 1 additional pound of fat.

This means if you overshoot by as little as 100 calories a meal (1/2 of a chocolate bar or 1/5 of a hamburger without cheese) and have three meals a day, you will gain a pound of fat every two weeks and a total of about 25 pounds over the year!

Figure 2 - How much is 500 calories of a given food?

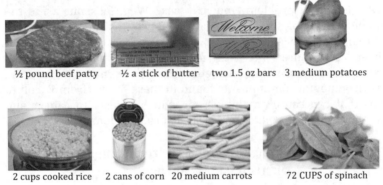

| ½ pound beef patty | ½ a stick of butter | two 1.5 oz bars | 3 medium potatoes |

| 2 cups cooked rice | 2 cans of corn | 20 medium carrots | 72 CUPS of spinach |

To make matters worse, we develop a dependence as well as a tolerance to this "dopamine hit."

Without even realizing it, we begin to rely on these foods to make us feel a certain way. There is a reason why we seek out pizza and brownies (higher calorie density and more dopamine released) and not cauliflower and wheatgrass (lower calorie density and less dopamine released) when we are feeling stressed or depressed. We are in fact drugging ourselves with the foods we eat (choosing more calorie-dense foods that stimulate more of a dopamine release). And, like addicts (which, in fact, is what we have unknowingly become) over time we develop tolerance, eventually seeking a greater high, which leads us to eat even more of these processed fatty foods.

Similar to a heroin addict who no longer feels pleasure from using the same drug dose, people living off fast food no longer feel pleasure from eating fruits and vegetables. You see this all of the time with children. Look at babies who have consumed nothing but breast milk for their first year of life. They then move on to plain cooked rice and enjoy that along with some pureed fruit. But once they get exposed to macaroni and cheese, try getting them to eat plain cooked cereal again; it's unlikely to happen without a fight. The idea here is that we eat the processed fast foods, we get our fix, we feel better, we start to wane, we go for our next fix (which is now the processed foods and not the fruits and vegetables) to relieve the "withdrawal" symptoms, we feel good again, and so on. And this is how we live day to day, meal to meal, stuck in the "Pleasure Trap."[9]

Take-home messages:

- **Your body is NOT flawed. This is not a problem resulting from defective genes, inability to portion control, or a propensity to emotionally eat.**

- **The problem lies in the environment we currently live in.**

- **We are inherently hard-wired to enjoy pleasurable experiences (like eating).**

- **The more calorie-dense a food is, the more pleasure we feel and the more dopamine is released.**

- **Our brain and our stomach work together to assess "calorie currency."**

- **The "caloric currency" system is accurate when eating natural whole foods.**

- **By eating natural whole foods we can avoid falling into the "Pleasure Trap."**

Chapter 2: Knowing Is Half the Battle

So, now we know why we do what we do. The next step is learning why we need to stop doing it. We, as Americans, are in danger of extinction; maybe not as a species (yet) and maybe not in the immediate future, but

> one by one we are prematurely digging our own graves.
> So much so, that for the first time in United States history,
> parents will likely outlive their children.[10]

And, although Americans may be living longer than ever, our life expectancy is shorter than that of most other industrialized nations, including Australia, France, Italy, Switzerland, Spain, Canada, Japan, and the United Kingdom.[11] As a matter of fact, according to the World Health Organization,

> "You die earlier and spend more time disabled
> if you're an American rather than
> a member of most other advanced countries."[12]

It is important to keep in perspective that this is so despite the fact that the United States has the highest per capita spending on healthcare.[13] So, we are spending more money on our health but are getting fatter and sicker and dying sooner. We don't know about you, but that doesn't sit well with us.

Which begs the question, where are we going wrong?

> Why are two-thirds of Americans overweight
> and of those, half obese? [4] Why is heart disease
> still our number one killer? And why is
> cancer still a close second?

Why do so many of us spend our last decades suffering a disease-laden life rather than thriving "until death do us take"? This is not nature taking its course, and this is certainly not the way things should be. In fact, we should be living a full, healthy, and vibrant life. Old age should mean a very slow and minimal decline of function, if at all. We should be living to see, and play with, our grandchildren and great-grandchildren; and not from a nursing home bed.

Our hearts should only ache when stricken with grief or sadness and not atherosclerotic plaque.

Cancer should be referred to when discussing astrology rather than chemotherapy or surgery.

And all of this should be accomplished without the latest medical procedures or pharmaceutical drugs.

We think you are probably getting our point by now and hope that most of you are excited to learn more. After all, who among us doesn't want to live a long, active, and healthy life? Who among us wouldn't want to avoid a medical procedure like a bypass, a mastectomy, chemotherapy or dialysis? Who wouldn't want to ditch their medications and their side effects, from high blood pressure pills to diabetic drugs to prescriptions for asthma or allergies? This is not only possible, it is probable, BUT it requires some effort. And the first order of business is to STOP DOING WHAT WE ARE DOING!

Our bodies are amazing machines, more advanced than anything technology or modern medicine has to offer us today.

Our hearts beat, our lungs breathe, our livers and kidneys filter, our stomachs digest, and this is happening automatically, concurrently, and continually within us. To attempt a comparison, try peeling a potato, talking on the telephone, standing on one foot, reading a magazine, and playing cards all at the same time. It's darn near, if not, impossible. Yet the trillions of cells in our bodies are continuously performing multiple complicated tasks, simultaneously, and with pinpoint precision all day, every day of our lives! And, for most of us, these cells are coming through for us even when we abuse them with poor nutrition, lack of exercise, inadequate sleep, and bad habits (like smoking). This is just one more example of the incredible resilience of the human body.

We need to stop taking our bodies for granted! We need to stop testing our body's ability to survive! We need to stop feeding ourselves junk! We need to stop poisoning ourselves with cigarettes, alcohol, and other drugs! We need to stop making excuses for our sedentary lifestyles, and we need to START embracing a change!

Take-home messages:

- **According to the World Health Organization, the United States ranks 22 out of 23 for industrialized nations' healthy life expectancy.**

- **Americans are spending more money on health but are getting fatter and sicker and dying sooner.**

- **For the first time in U.S. history, parents will likely outlive their children.**

- **Two-thirds of Americans are overweight, and of those, half are obese.**

- **Our bodies are amazing machines, more advanced than anything technology or modern medicine has to offer us today.**

Chapter 3: Embracing a Change

We are making progress. We now know why we do what we do and why we need to stop doing it. In this chapter we begin to learn how. There is certainly no shortage of information on how to get healthy and feel better. We are bombarded daily with media ads, commercials, billboards, and pamphlets advertising the new "expert" on the block and his/her latest miracle cure. The biggest culprits in this wealth, *oops*, we mean health, industry are the medical and pharmaceutical companies. It would be nice to believe these businesses had our best interest in mind, but that is difficult to do when

> iatrogenic (caused by the medical system)
> deaths are the third leading cause of death in
> this country after heart attacks and cancer![15]

In 1995, a report in JAMA (Journal of the American Medical Association) stated that "Over a million patients are injured in U.S. hospitals each year, and approximately 280,000 die annually as a result of injuries. Therefore, the iatrogenic death rate dwarfs the annual automobile accident mortality rate of 45,000 and accounts for more deaths than all other accidents combined."[16]

Yes, these incidents are considered "accidents" and may be forgivable by some; but what about the boldface lies told to us by the medical and pharmaceutical companies? Does anyone remember the Vioxx scandal that revealed that Merck (the company that made Vioxx) knew their product had dangerous side effects (specifically heart risks) but pushed it into the market anyway?[17] What about the Hormone Replacement Therapy (HRT) debacle? HRT was initially prescribed to decrease menopausal symptoms as well as protect from osteoporosis and heart disease but was then found to increase cancer and impede the accuracy of mammograms (thus interfering with early detection), and promote (not prevent) heart disease![18,19,20] Or, how about the fact that

pharmaceutical companies influence "thought leaders"
or experts in a particular medical field and use them to help
convince other physicians to use their drugs.[21]

According to a JAMA article, "59% of authors of clinical practice guidelines (these are the recommendations doctors follow in treating their patients) had relationships with companies whose drugs were considered in the guidelines they authored."[22] In the 2004 updated cholesterol guidelines (the recommendations our doctors use to treat us), eight out of nine authors had financial ties to statin drug companies.[23] Is it any wonder then why we use statin drugs as our number one cholesterol-lowering medication? One final example for you to ponder, not from lack of material but because we don't wish to completely overwhelm you, is the issue of the medical journals (where physicians look for their guidance in treating patients). Currently, 75% of clinical trials published in the best medical journals (NEJM, JAMA, and Lancet) are commercially funded.[24] An article in JAMA reported that commercially funded trials were five times (or 500%!) more likely to recommend an experimental drug as their treatment of choice. The conclusion from this study was,

"Trials funded by for-profit organizations may be
more positive due to biased interpretation of trial
results. Readers should carefully evaluate
whether conclusions in randomized trials
are supported by data."[25]

The New England Journal of Medicine looked at the 25% of studies still conducted at Universities, our last bastion of hope for unbiased, academic, evidence-based research. They found that 50% of contracts in ACADEMIC research allowed drug companies to write the first draft of the article! Even more astonishing, 25% of the contracts allowed the drug companies to put in their data tables instead of the tables prepared by the original authors.[26] Other interesting statistics in the article above include: 80% of the studies paid for by the drug firm manufacturing the tested drug come out positive (meaning they show the drug is beneficial), but only 30% of the studies paid for by drug companies testing a competitor's drug come out positive. Furthermore, drug companies have been known to end studies early if they see the results are heading in the wrong direction to avoid having to report their findings to the FDA (Food and Drug Administration).[27] Again, this is just the tip of the iceberg.

So, are we saying you can't trust your doctors? Or, that medication is never appropriate? **No, not at all!** What we are saying is that

you need to be vigilant about your healthcare because there is a lot of misinformation out there.

So much so, that even doctors get duped. They read the medical journals and they follow the guidelines; but that is not always necessarily in the patient's best interest. And this is because, as we have learned, there are a lot of biases that affect research outcomes— yes, even medical research, as you have just witnessed. And when we do need medical care from the medical industry, it would be in our best interest to be sure that we have truly exhausted all safer options before taking this risk. But, don't start panicking yet. This does not mean that everything you hear is wrong, it just means that you shouldn't believe everything you hear. As H. Gilbert Welch, MD (author of the book *Should I Be Tested For Cancer*) recommends,

"Have a healthy skepticism." Question...question...and then question some more; this becomes your job.

Our job, then, becomes sharing the answers we have discovered by asking such questions ourselves. Furthermore, our intent is to provide you with information that is evidence-based, medically prudent, and ethically sound. Often this involves reviewing the medical literature with our patients. Sometimes part of the treatment includes medications and, occasionally, even recommendations for procedures. But more often than not, we will ask you to go back to the basics. And, in doing so, our recommendations will build on assets you already have: your body, your time, and your investment in your health.

In essence, our program is designed to help you achieve *your* optimum health and as such invites you to create *your* own path at *your* own pace. What we offer are suggestions based on scientific evidence that we have gathered over the years.

We have learned that most people can benefit immensely from diet and lifestyle modifications.

How much you gain depends on how quickly and how intensely you choose to transition. Keep in mind that the name of the game is long-term, lifetime, and forever, so this is not a race.

We believe health lies on a continuum where one extreme is disease (0%, see Figure 3) and the other is optimal wellness (100%, see Figure 3). In other words, someone who has a heart attack today wasn't healthy yesterday; rather they just moved close enough to 0% on the continuum to be noticed. Living between 90-100% on the Optimum Health Continuum, for most people, is ideal for promoting optimal health. Note that the Optimum Health Continuum is a scale used at Exsalus to treat patients in a comprehensive manner by incorporating medical, physical, and psychological factors that we believe must be addressed to achieve optimum health.

Figure 3 - Sample Optimum Health Continuum

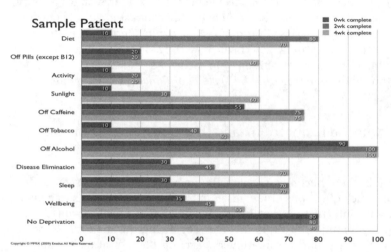

Is there a benefit to being at 100% over 90%? Can some of us be comfortably healthy at 70% or 80%? Will some of us live to be 100+ at 50%? The collective answer to these questions is possibly, but as an individual this is not where your focus should lie. Does it matter if your neighbor smokes like a chimney at 85 years old or that your Aunt Sally lived to be 110 years old? No. Most of you know that in the former case, living next door to someone has no bearing on your health, and in the latter case genetics plays a minimal role, if any. There is a popular saying in the field that states,

"Genetics loads the gun but environment pulls the trigger."

What we inherit—the good and the bad—is just one component of our make-up. What we do with those genes is what really counts.

Our goal should be to thrive not just survive.

In other words, what matters is:

1) What you have done to your health and your body up to this point (for many of us that includes a disease-promoting diet and lifestyle),
2) Where that leaves you on the continuum, and
3) What changes (if any) you need to make from here.

And that is where our program comes in. The Exsalus Health Program is intended to take you from where you are to where you want to be, with each step tailored to your needs and set to your pace. Moreover, it is flexible and dynamic so that as your needs and obstacles change, so can the program.

You are probably wondering at this point, why you should listen to us. Great question! The answer is DON'T! Listen to yourself. Are you satisfied with your health? Do you feel good most of the time? Are you as energetic as you would like to be? Have you attained your goal weight without feeling hunger pangs and/or deprivation? Are you certain you aren't developing heart disease and cancer too early to be detected at this point? If you answered "yes" to all of these questions, congratulations and keep doing what you are doing. But, if you answered "no" to ANY of these questions then read on because we just might have a better solution for you.

Most of you have heard the famous saying,

>"Give a man a fish and you feed him for a day;
>teach him how to fish and you feed him for a lifetime."

We want to ensure you reach your goals whether they are losing weight, reversing disease, recapturing your lost health and vitality, or all of the above. Our plan is thus designed to teach you "to fish" by:

1) Providing you with knowledge that will make you a more informed participant in your healthcare,
2) Helping you determine where you want to be on the health continuum, and
3) Providing you with simple and easy tips to get you there.

Our hope is not that you follow us blindly but that you consider what we have to say and give us an opportunity to show you the data. We are confident you will find, as we did, that this program not only makes sense but is doable and gets results.

Take-home messages:

- Be vigilant about your healthcare; there is a lot of misinformation out there.

- Iatrogenic (caused by the medical system) deaths are the THIRD leading cause of death in this country after heart attacks and cancer.

- The iatrogenic death rate accounts for more deaths than ALL other accidents combined.

- Pharmaceutical companies influence "thought leaders" to help sell their drugs.

- "Genetics loads the gun but environment pulls the trigger."

- Health lies on a continuum.

Chapter 4: A New Paradigm for Health

There is no doubt that, for most of you, the Exsalus Health Program will attain the results you desire. But in order to be successful, we must work together. As we have already stated, our job is to provide you with the knowledge and the skills that you need to make a permanent and positive lifestyle change. Your job is to be open to our new paradigm for health and health-care.

Charles Darwin said, "It is not the strongest of the species that survive, nor the most intelligent, but the one most responsive to change."

We are due for a change in our healthcare system.

The old model is not working because it leaves too many people sick, fat, and dependent on medications and procedures that cause too much harm and not enough benefit. It is time to commit to something new, and no time is better than the present.

So, what are we proposing? We believe healthcare must be comprehensive. The World Health Organization knew and stated this over 60 years ago when they defined optimal health as "a state of complete physical, mental, and social well-being."[28] True healthcare must incorporate nutrition, clean habits, sleep, exercise, relaxation, and a social support structure. Someone who is lean but smokes is not healthy. Nor is someone who is otherwise well but takes sleeping pills every night to get some rest.

Optimal health is "a state of complete physical, mental, and social well-being."

Our current healthcare model is not built to address this need for comprehensive care. A ten-minute visit with the doctor barely scratches the surface of a chief complaint, much less tackles any underlying issues or implements support structures for significant lifestyle changes. Is it any wonder then that these visits often result in quick-fix treatments aimed at controlling symptoms rather than identifying causes? Or, that we have become a society dependant on medication to feel "normal?" No, not at all. And true, this system makes the numbers in the medical chart look better (cholesterol, blood pressure, blood glucose, etc.) but does it actually make patients healthier? Again, no, not at all! Bringing your cholesterol down with a pill but continuing your same unhealthy lifestyle will still lead to heart disease. Controlling your blood sugar with medications doesn't get rid of your diabetes. In fact, attaining normal numbers as a result of taking pills often gives people a false sense of security and has been associated with significant risk of illness and death. In other words,

> normal numbers achieved with pills
> do NOT equate to the same health
> as normal numbers without pills
> (such as achieving normal blood pressure
> through a healthy diet and lifestyle).

For example, men (40-59 years old) had a 21% risk of death from stroke over 3 years and a 20% risk of death from heart attack over 3 years even if their blood pressure was reduced from 183/114 down to 149/91 with medication. Compare that to a 1% risk of death in people who were un-medicated with a blood pressure of 133/80.[29] We always tell our patients that normal numbers don't mean normal health if you are manipulating those numbers with pills. The pills you take manage some of the numbers associated with your diseases, but they don't help you overcome or cure them. The bottom line comes down to what are you most worried about: your numbers or your health?

Manage your health, not your numbers.

Optimal health should be about eliminating quick fixes and identifying the sources of your ailments. Only in this manner can you truly hope to rid yourself of illness. The difficulty is time and the challenge is taking the time.

What appeared over years will not disappear in one night.

Moreover, time is essential in allowing both doctor and patient to identify and address the obstacles currently preventing a healthy diet and lifestyle change. This is a tough concept to embrace in a world that seeks out and thrives on immediate gratification, as it goes against the core of our dopamine-pleasure cycle discussed in Chapter 1. We never want to exchange pleasure for pain, even temporarily. As a matter of fact, our bodies are hard-wired to avoid pain and conserve energy at all costs. No wonder, in our medical care, we turn to procedures and medications over lifestyle modifications—the return is almost instantaneous, albeit often transient. Our personal lives are no different. We live in a society that measures our value by our productivity, material possessions, and financial successes. In essence,

we are rewarded (a pleasurable experience) for "burning the candle at both ends."

And although we believe this gains us status, happiness, and worth, in reality, it only leads to premature and rapid extinction.

The new health paradigm we are proposing requires a suspension of life as you know it today. By that we mean replacing the life that is not rewarding you with the health and happiness you desire and deserve. We are asking you to do something that for many of you will be very scary: return to "the basics," a place where you can trust your bodies. This is an impossible feat with the American diet and lifestyle—an artificial environment in which our bodies cannot thrive. Furthermore, we are asking you to enter the turtle race, where patience is the rewarded virtue (remember the analogy of learning a new language, discussed in our introduction). It may not feel good at first, it may even be uncomfortable, but slow and steady will win your race and eventually you will feel fantastic.

Take-home messages:

- **Optimal health is "a state of complete physical, mental, and social well-being."**
- **Normal numbers DO NOT mean normal health IF you are manipulating those numbers with pills.**
- **Optimal health should be about eliminating quick fixes and identifying the actual sources of your ailments.**
- **"Burning the candle at both ends" leads to premature and rapid extinction.**

Chapter 5: The Exsalus Challenge

Exsalus Health & Wellness Center challenges you to enter the race. Your progress will be individual and driven by your goals and motivation. Remember your end goal as you begin your transition to health: This is a commitment you are making to yourself and your loved ones for the rest of your life. As such,

pick a pace that you can stick with, that moves you closer to optimal health but doesn't leave you deprived, miserable, and eventually non-compliant.

If you move to the right from 50% and find you need to live at 75% for a while then pat yourself on the back for making such wonderful progress. Stay there until you are ready to move forward.

50%   75%

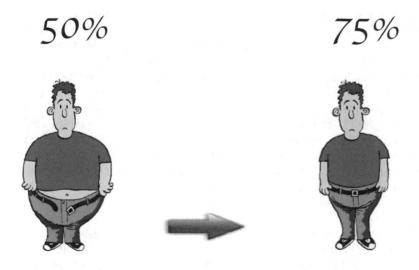

There is no benefit to jumping from 50% to 90% for three months, deciding that the new change is too drastic and returning to live at 50%. Especially if this squanders the opportunity for you to possibly live at 75%.

$$50\% \rightarrow 90\% \rightarrow 50\%$$

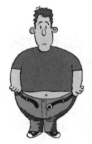 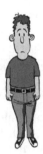 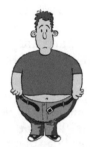

You may even decide that your end-goal is 75%, and that works too! The point is that the plan is flexible and geared toward improving your overall health. Going from 30% to 50%, 70%, or 90% is moving in the **right** direction and that is what you should be striving for. Sometimes, jumping in 100% to see how good it feels to be healthy is fun too, so choose what works best for you. An analogy would be traveling from Los Angeles to New York. You can fly, drive, or walk understanding that there are advantages and disadvantages to each mode of transportation. The goal, however, is to head east and you have to decide what time frame works best for you. For many of our patients this process is dynamic. Their pace changes as they become more familiar with their new lifestyle and as each positive change builds on the previous.

If you are questioning the value of taking this challenge, remember that this is an investment for yourself and your family. After all, don't you want to be around (not only surviving but thriving) for the next 30, 40, or 50+ years? Wouldn't it be great to be free of heart disease, high cholesterol, cancer, and diabetes? How about achieving your trim weight without diets, restrictions, and deprivation? Or, being free of the constraints (money, time, and side effects) of medications? What about being able to make everyday your best, your healthiest, your most energetic, and your happiest? Sound tempting? Well, this could be you. Moreover, this should be you.

If you decide that at this point you are not quite ready to take this challenge, we commend you for being honest. The truth is that this program will only work if you are ready and therefore committed to making the necessary changes. Those of you who aren't there yet, keep this book somewhere easily accessible to re-visit when you are ready.

For those of you who are ready, congratulations! You have just made the greatest investment in your life and we are certain that you will not regret your decision.

So, what are we asking of you? One month, that is it. BUT, in order to be successful, you must make the commitment to adhere strictly to the program for that month. What does that mean? Well,

the "program" will be different for every one of you and, again, will depend on where you are on the Optimum Health Continuum, where you would like to be, and the pace of your transition.

The most important step for you is deciding how much you can realistically do, for this one month, and then sticking to that plan 100%. For some of you, this may involve making modest changes, while for others the changes may be drastic. And, of course, the degree of change to which you commit will directly correlate with the intensity of your results.

Those of you making the bigger changes will see bigger results. BUT, if you follow your plan 100%, there is no doubt you will see yourself move to the right along the Optimum Health Continuum. And that should be your number one priority,

not how fast you move but that you are moving in the **right** direction at a pace that works for you.

We cannot emphasize this enough: TO BE SUCCESSFUL YOU MUST CHOOSE A REALISTIC PACE FOR YOU; even if that means it will take you several weeks, months, or years to attain your final goal. Too often we have seen gunners decide they are going straight to the top or to 100%. They might manage this for one, two, three, or even six months as they continue to see and be motivated by positive results. But, eventually and inevitably, they begin to feel deprived, their new lifestyle becomes a miserable diet, they become unhappy and begin to have cravings, and the next thing you know they are wolfing down anything they can get their hands on (hamburgers, French fries, cream puffs, fried chicken, chocolate bars, etc.). We have witnessed the detrimental effects of this deprivation-binge cycle all too often, and we can advise you with absolute certainty that you do not want to fall victim to it. So, be good to yourself, be honest with yourself, and prepare for long-term success.

> Make this change about adopting a new lifestyle
> rather than reverting to a temporary quick fix.

Move along the health continuum gradually so that you have time to acclimate and catch your breath before you continue on. And, if you do decide to jump in at 100% be mindful of how you feel, monitor your cravings, and note any feelings of deprivation. If you find that you have not yet learned the tools to satisfy your cravings in a healthy way and/or that your level of deprivation is escalating, you may want to go down to 90% or 80% for a while. This temporary shift may be essential to keep you on the program as you gain new and necessary skills to handle cravings and deprivation.

Again, this is analogous to learning a new language. Some of you may feel you are ready to immerse yourself in a language after two or three weeks of instruction (similar to jumping to 100% on the Exsalus Health Program). But, once immersed, you may find that you would benefit greatly from taking time to learn a few more words, conjugate a few more verbs, and build a few more sentences. The same theory applies to the Exsalus Health Program. Having said that, our intention is not to discourage you from jumping in 100%; on the contrary, we applaud that drive and determination. Based on the science alone, 100% compliance makes the most sense. But there is also an art to long-term success, which has nothing to do with the science.

> So, while 100% compliance may bring faster changes,
> the long-term results are more important
> than the speed in which you achieve those results.

Often when patients are pushed too far, they quit; some never to be seen again and others to return when their illnesses have become so grave that they are facing the choice between expensive and harmful medications, extremely invasive procedures, or inevitable death. This then becomes a balancing act between pushing you out of your comfort zone to learn this new language without pushing you so far that we never see or hear from you again. Be aware of this dynamic and in doing so remain realistic about what you can do so that you will be able to keep it up for a long, long time.

As with all general recommendations, you hammer them home, you make sure everyone understands them and is on board, and then you introduce the exceptions. And there are always exceptions! In this case, it would be those of you with very serious or end-stage diseases that are time sensitive. Some examples include, but are not limited to, a new cancer diagnosis, severe and debilitating arthritis, a history of multiple heart attacks, and/or a doctor prescribing bypass surgery. Those of you that fall into these, or similar, categories have aggressive disease that must be met with equally aggressive treatment. Under these circumstances we generally do not have the luxury of running a turtle's race. Nor can we afford to live anywhere on the health continuum other than at optimal health. This is because we need our bodies to function at maximal capacity to battle our particular illness, especially in its most aggressive stages.

To emphasize this point, imagine discovering a fire is headed toward your home versus waking up to a fire destroying your home. In the former case, you may have time to gather important or sentimental personal items before leaving. You may even choose to stay put, in the house or near the house, hoping that the fire will be squelched before it reaches you. The same applies for those of you who have mild to moderate disease or who just want to improve your health. You have the time to slowly and steadily climb the health continuum and the choice to stay put (temporarily or permanently) along the way. But, if you are in the midst of the fire, you must leave your house immediately and get as far away as you can. In this case, there is no time to gather memoirs and no choice but to escape. In the same manner, for those of you battling a severe illness, time is of the essence. You must hurry to your final destination (in this case optimal health) and get there without making any stops. As such, the "program" for you would be accelerated and a bit more rigid but very doable and well worth it, especially with the right support and guidance.

Also, keep in mind that although we are "racing for the cure," if you will, the rigidity of this regimen is temporary. The intention is to get you to the strongest, healthiest place you can be to battle your illness. However, once you have optimized your health and managed your disease, some of you will be able to loosen the reins and return to a more flexible plan if needed. How flexible it becomes depends on your particular disease. It is only natural to test your boundaries and limits but do so carefully as it is a slippery slope.

So far, we have spent a lot of time asking things of you. Now, the time has come for us to share with you the health-promoting benefits you can begin to expect from committing to our challenge.

Take-home messages:

- **Remember you are learning a new language, the language of optimum health.**

- **To be successful you must choose a realistic pace.**

- **Pick a pace that you can stick with, that moves you closer to optimal health but doesn't leave you deprived, miserable and, eventually, non-compliant.**

- **Make this change about adopting a new lifestyle rather than a temporary quick fix.**

- **Sometimes a small shift may be essential to keep you on the program as you gain new and necessary skills to handle cravings and deprivation.**

- **This is a commitment you are making to yourself and your loved ones for the rest of your life.**

Chapter 6: The Numerous Benefits

In this chapter, we discuss the numerous benefits that can be expected by committing to the Exsalus Health Program. Notice we don't specify who will benefit; that is because

> ### we are confident that ANYONE and EVERYONE
> ### can benefit from our program.

The question then is not, "Can I benefit?" but, "How **much** can I benefit?" Ultimately, as we have discussed in the previous chapters, the amount of benefit will depend on you and your level of commitment and participation.

So, what are some of the health-promoting benefits you can expect?[1]

1) **First, is the reversal of debilitating chronic diseases** including, but not limited to, heart disease, cancer, diabetes, stroke, and chronic fatigue. Following the Exsalus Health Program can result in decreased cholesterol and atherosclerosis (plaque build-up in your arteries), reduction or elimination of tumor growth and prevention of tumor development, and management and stabilization of blood sugar levels and blood pressures. As an added bonus, vitality improves and pain levels are significantly diminished or disappear altogether.

2) **Second, is weight loss.** Participants of the program can expect to shed excess pounds without restricting or depriving themselves of tasty and delicious meals. How much and how quickly you lose your weight, again, depends on the pace you choose. The closer you get to optimal health on the health continuum, the more likely you will be to achieve your ideal slim and trim weight. The reason this works is that as you

---

[1] These are typical results for most patients who have achieved 90%-100% on their Optimum Health Continuum (OHC) parameters.

move to the right of the Optimum Health Continuum, you are developing healthier practices. These include making better food choices, sleeping better, exercising, and eliminating bad habits (such as smoking). All of these components positively affect weight loss and health, so it is no wonder that in combination they are that much more powerful.

3) **Third, is the ability to discontinue medications.** Most of you will be able to reduce or eliminate your medications for high blood pressure, type II diabetes, arthritis, indigestion, reflux, and constipation, among other things. Imagine the freedom that will come with being healthy without having to depend on pills, without having to worry about paying for them, without being limited by their schedule, and without having to endure their side effects. (Please note you should NOT alter your medication regimens without physician supervision.)

4) **Next, is improvement in vigor, vitality, and overall well-being within DAYS of starting the program.** You will shed those feelings of fatigue, heaviness, and mental cloudiness and they will be replaced by energy, agility, and clarity. In addition, rather than crashing after a meal, feeling sluggish at best, you will be invigorated.

5) **Finally, you can save thousands of dollars per year in food and health care costs.** Sound too good to be true? Let's take a closer look, beginning with research that has shown that adopting healthier eating habits can save you as much as $2000 to $4500 a year.[30] Add to that the thousands of dollars per year you can save just by stopping five of the most commonly used medications (for cholesterol, high blood pressure, osteoporosis, reflux, and arthritis). Moreover, many of you have bought into the need for taking supplements to enhance your diets. Unfortunately, not all of these supplements are necessary and, in fact, taking some of them may be doing us more harm than good. (For more information on supplements, see Chapter 13.) Discontinuing such supplementation may not only be beneficial to your health but it may further save you hundreds to thousands of dollars per year. Additional savings will result from: fewer visits to the doctor (as a result of overall better health), not needing to join diet programs (that cost a lot and don't work for most of us in the long run), and not requiring medical procedures and their expensive recovery programs (from angioplasty to bypass to liposuction).

The bottom line is that the Exsalus Health Program can take you from diseased to healthy, from overweight to trim, from lethargic to energetic, and from discouraged to hopeful. And all this can happen while saving you money! Sound enticing? We think so. So, without further ado, let us introduce the Exsalus Health Program.

Take-home messages:

- **It is not, "Can you benefit?" but "How much can you benefit?"**
- **Benefits of the Exsalus Health Program:**
  - **Reversal of chronic disease (heart disease, cancer, diabetes, stroke, arthritis, fibromyalgia, chronic fatigue, etc.)**
  - **Weight loss without restricting or being deprived**
  - **Elimination of medications (blood pressure, cholesterol, etc.)**
  - **Increased energy, vigor, vitality, and overall well-being**
  - **Savings of thousands of dollars per year in food and healthcare costs**

Chapter 7: The Exsalus Health Program

The Exsalus Health Program is straightforward. This plan is evidence-based, resulting from years of research, both clinical and in the field. We are fortunate to walk in the footsteps of pioneer greats such as John McDougall, MD, T. Colin Campbell, PhD., Caldwell B. Esselstyn, Jr., MD, Neal Barnard, MD, Joel Fuhrman, MD, and Doug Lisle, PhD. These scholars and clinicians have dedicated their lives to investigating, studying, confirming, and compiling the copious evidence available to us today. Thanks to their hard work, there is no shortage of data supporting the Exsalus Health Program.

Guided by their knowledge and their templates, we have compiled a nutrition and lifestyle model that we are confident will work for you. In addition, we have included as part of the appendices, for your convenience, a small workbook for you to fill out as you navigate through the Exsalus Health Program. The workbook is intended to help you implement the practical portion of this diet and lifestyle. In other words, we can talk until we are blue in the face (or in this case write until we are out of ink), but that pales in comparison to the progress you will make if you roll up your sleeves and get your hands dirty. So, take advantage of the resources available throughout, especially in the back of this book, as they will prove to be very useful tools in building and strengthening your fluency in this new language of optimum health.

The remainder of this chapter will give you an overview of this model. The following chapters will fill in the details.

Our program revolves around two key findings. The first is that,

there are no health benefits
to eating animal products,

short of a famine where food is scarce. The second is that,

people are healthier on an oil-free
(not fat-free), whole foods, plant-based diet.

Specifically, in switching over to a plant-based diet, most people are able to reverse their heart disease, decrease their cholesterol, lower their blood pressure, cure type II diabetes (or significantly improve type I diabetes), effortlessly reduce their weight, and eliminate their chronic and nagging aches and pains. In addition, as their general wellbeing improves, they gain vitality, agility, energy, and happiness.

So, are we saying you have to eat a 100% plant-based diet? No, what we are saying is that,

the more plant-based your diet is,
the healthier you will be.

For some of you, in the initial transition stages, you may begin by addressing your vegetable and fruit deficiencies. This may mean adding a helping of vegetables to your steak and potatoes or having an apple with your chocolate chip cookies (see Table 1, example 1). In this case, we would recommend that you eat your vegetables and your apple first and then consume the rest of your meal. This serves two purposes: 1) it ensures that you will eat the healthier options, and 2) it allows you to fill up on these healthier foods before continuing with the less healthy choices. If you were questioning the benefits of these small changes, keep in mind that even adding one apple a day was shown to decrease all sorts of cancers, including cancer of the mouth, throat, breast, colon, kidney, and ovary.[31] Furthermore, the apple peels were shown to be particularly beneficial in women with the more difficult to treat, estrogen-receptor-negative breast cancer.[32]

For others, you may start substituting healthier foods for less healthy foods. This may involve substituting a bean burrito for your usual chicken or beef burrito or it may involve choosing a soymilk-based ice cream instead of the dairy version (see Table 1, example 2). Are we saying that you can eat all the soy ice cream you want? Not by a long shot. But, we are saying that, based on the science, if you are going to eat ice cream, selecting the non-dairy (soy, rice, etc.) variety over the dairy is a healthier choice.[33]

And still for others, it may mean adopting a diet rich in fruits, vegetables, grains, and legumes with minimal to no processed foods (see Table 1, example 3). In this manner, you most readily eliminate unhealthy foods replacing them with healthy options, while simultaneously flooding your body with these nutrient-packed foods.

Table 1 - Examples of transitioning your diet.

Example 1	Adding a serving of vegetables to your steak and potatoes OR having an apple with your chocolate chip cookie. OR
Example 2	Substituting a bean burrito for your usual chicken or beef burrito OR choosing soymilk ice cream instead of the dairy version. OR
Example 3	Adopting a diet rich in fruits, vegetables, grains, and legumes with minimal to no processed foods.

The decision will be individual and based on the pace you have chosen to move along the health continuum.

> Keep in mind that the "cleaner" your diet is—
> meaning the more natural whole foods
> (fruits, vegetables, whole grains, and legumes)
> that you incorporate—the higher up you will move
> on the continuum (closer to 100% on the OHC).

Having said this, we will re-emphasize the importance of MAINTAINING YOUR PACE, because achieving long-term compliance will be the key to your success. So, although example 3 (see Table 1) is the healthiest choice based on the science and will move you much higher up the continuum than examples 1 or 2, if you are not ready or cannot commit to that change then it is not a goal you should be striving for right now.

Understand too that your pace may increase as you are transitioning. There are few things more motivating than positive reinforcement. As you continue to climb up the health continuum, you will not only be feeling healthier but you will be looking healthier. You will be hearing things like, "WOW, you look fantastic, what's different?" or "You've lost a lot of weight, what are you doing?" Your doctors may be pleasantly surprised to see your blood pressure decreasing, your cholesterol going down, and your blood sugar under better control. Most importantly, you will look at yourself and see a new radiance, a new confidence, and a new vitality that will motivate you to continue on your path. It may even inspire you to challenge yourself further and step it up a notch along your individual continuum.

To help guide you, we have included a Food Continuum for you to reference.[34] (For a more detailed explanation please refer to Appendix B.)

Figure 4 – Food Continuum[34]

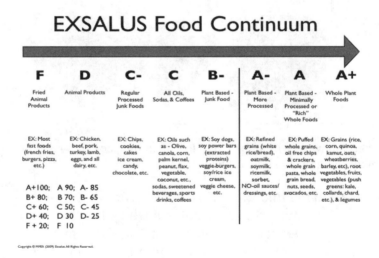

The ultimate goal is to live in the A range.

Why not A+, you may ask? Although A+ is a superior diet, it is, at best, harder to maintain and at worst unrealistic to achieve long-term. We find that many patients striving for that goal or even attaining it, end up feeling deprived and unsatisfied. This dissatisfaction eventually leads to bingeing, straying, or abandoning the program altogether.

Those are not the results we are looking for. So, we feel that living in the A range (which still requires a significant foundation of A+ foods) affords you the most flexibility while still ultimately preserving your health.

There are many ways to stay within an A range. The most obvious is eating 100% of your foods from the A and A+ column. But, you could also average an A over an entire day or over a specific meal. In this case, you might choose to eat 75% of your meal (or meals for the day) from the A+ column and 25% from the C column or 50% from the A+ column, 30% from the A column, and 20% from the B- column. The combinations are endless, but we think you get the point.

Now, having said that, you may not be able to jump from where you are to an A diet. WE DON'T EXPECT YOU TO! (Unless, of course, you fall into one of the extreme cases we mentioned as exceptions at the end of Chapter 5.) That is why this program, for most of you, will be a transition to a healthier you; more like a journey rather than a quick fix. As such, some of you will be going from an F to a C average, and that will be a remarkable accomplishment. Others will go from a C to a B average, etc.

> ## Keep your eye on moving higher up on the Food Continuum[34], not how much or how fast you do so.

Always keep in mind that the closer you get to the A range the healthier you will be BUT only if your well-being (by this we mean your level of stress, your overall mood, your energy, etc.) parallels your diet changes (see Figure 5).

Figure 5 – Sample Patient Optimum Health Continuum

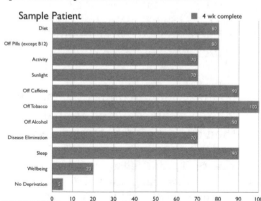

What we mean by this is that you are not achieving optimal health (which includes mental, emotional, and physical health) if your diet is at an 80% but your well-being is at a 20% and your deprivation is through the roof.

Figure 6 – Frustration resulting from decreased well-being and increased deprivation.

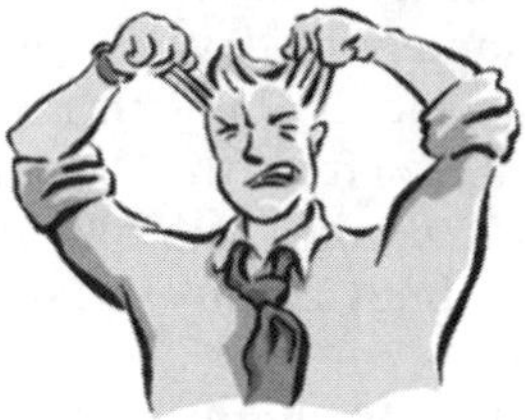

In this scenario (see Figures 5 and 6), more often than not, patients give up entirely. Now, maybe their deprivation and stress are lowered but their diet returns to 30% (we are being generous), their diseases reappear, and as a result they feel terrible and their well-being suffers once again. These are not the results we are hoping to achieve.

So, take a look at the Food Continuum[34] and give yourself a goal for this week. If you are at an F and there is no way you can give up those fried foods, then for this week try to limit your intake of these foods. You can do this by either limiting yourself to only one fried meal a day while making the rest of your meals healthy choices OR you could have your meals with a vegetable or fruit dish such as a large bean and veggie salad (vegetable or fruit with no dressing or oil-free/fat-free dressing) or a vegetable and bean soup. You can even try to just add one oil-free, plant-based recipe per week to your growing arsenal of healthy foods. The first week you might try to tackle a healthy, oil-free, plant-based lasagna (see Appendix I). The next week could be an oil-free, Asian stir-fry (see Appendix I). If the dish doesn't taste good one week then try a new recipe the next. Eventually you will build up a large repertoire of healthy, oil-free, plant-based dishes from which to choose.

One steadfast and uncompromising rule is:
have the vegetable, fruit, or grain dish first,
then have the rest of your meal.

Again, this is because 1) this ensures you will eat those more nutritious foods, and 2) this will allow you to fill up on the healthier choices, leaving less room for the unhealthier ones.

Maybe you are at an F and are willing to jump to a C average but can't completely give up the animal products. Okay, then base your diet around the A+ and A foods (vegetables, fruits, legumes, and grains) and include a very small portion of the D foods (animal products). In this manner, you average a C for that meal.

The most important thing to remember in using the Food Continuum[34] is to ADD; make sure you ADD in your whole foods to every meal (your fruits, vegetables, legumes, and grains).

And, make sure that you eat these foods before indulging in more fatty, plant-based dishes, animal products, or processed foods.

Ideally, you want to think of a 3-Phase Eating Plan or simply having your meal in 3 courses.

The first course is your "weight loss medicine and multivitamin" consisting of your vegetables (or fruit for breakfast).

Your goal should be to have one big bowl of these foods; they can be raw, steamed, sautéed in an oil-free sauce, etc. Note, this course should NOT be skipped.

The second course is your "filler" and incorporates whole foods (foods that are not manipulated or highly processed).

Foods to be considered in course 2 are: brown rice, potatoes, corn, oats, quinoa, bulgur, squash, legumes, etc. For example, brown rice and beans, potatoes and salsa, a quinoa salad with corn, green onions, and currants. The combinations are limited only by your imagination. Again, remember you want to have a decent sized bowl of these foods prior to moving on to course 3. In order to succeed long-term, you MUST include this second course.

The third course is optional and includes processed, healthy and/or more fatty plant foods.

These include: whole-grain breads or pastas, corn tortillas, whole-grain chips or crackers, non-dairy milks, lasagna, pizza, burritos/enchiladas. This course is optional, as filling up on course 2 would suffice. However, if course 3 is eaten, it should be a much smaller portion of your overall meal. The beauty is that if you incorporate this 3-course or 3-phase meal plan, the third course will naturally be smaller because you will not be as hungry, having already consumed generous portions of courses 1 and 2. "Richer" plant foods, such as nuts, seeds, avocados, olives, or soy, should be included in this category as well and when used, if used at all, should be a "seasoning" to your meal rather than a main dish. For example, you can sprinkle nuts on your vegetable noodle dish (but don't eat a bowl of nuts) or you can add some guacamole to your enchilada (but don't just eat an avocado).

Although this may seem like a hassle at the beginning, it is a very important step in learning this new language of optimum health. For those of you that would be helped by a gimmick, find one that you can adhere to. For example, the broccoli and sweet potato diet, the cauliflower and quinoa diet, the greens, beans, and brown rice diet, etc. In other words, no matter what you choose to eat, promise yourself that you will have a bowl of each of these foods before EVERY meal (and hold yourself accountable for doing so). This is obviously not necessary but it does help to retrain your approach to eating so that you will no longer be having just pizza for dinner. Rather, you will be having broccoli and sweet potatoes (or whatever your gimmick happens to be) AND THEN a slice of pizza for dinner.

> Once eating this way becomes second nature,
> you can put all the food onto one plate and
> eat everything altogether rather than
> breaking it up into three distinct courses.

The reason for not doing this at the beginning is because most people who have broccoli, rice, and dumplings on their plate will eat the dumplings first, the rice next, and then if they feel like it, might nibble at the broccoli (although by that time, for most people, dessert will be calling their name and will never fail to look more appetizing than broccoli!) So, do yourself a favor and begin your re-training by mindfully having 3 courses. This is analogous to learning a new dance; you begin one step at a time, and when you have mastered the individual steps, you put the dance together. Note that you may add sauces (oil-free and low-fat) to enhance the taste of any course, just be sure to use these as seasonings.

While you are learning this new language, or new dance, always remember to monitor your deprivation. This does not mean to run back to your old foods and habits at the first sign of deprivation...not by a long shot! But, it does mean that these feelings must be acknowledged and addressed. Although your first instinct may be to panic, it is important to remember that most changes are challenging and may leave us longing for familiar comforts (whatever they may be). As such,

cravings and deprivation are very normal feelings,

especially when encountering the unknown, in this case unfamiliar new dishes and new ways of cooking. The key here is to acknowledge and recognize rather than suppress this discomfort as a natural stage of change. The next step is to identify why we are feeling deprived. What are we craving? Is it a certain taste or texture? Is it an association we have made to a particular food or experience (e.g., eating ice cream to alleviate our depression and elevate our mood, consuming a tub of buttered popcorn at the movies, or having a cup of coffee to get our juices flowing in the morning)? Or, are we just hungry, and would the cravings/deprivation go away if we had something to eat?

The final step is to:

figure out how to address and/or incorporate these desires into your new lifestyle.

For example, if your cravings arise mostly when you are hungry and you do not have an opportunity to sit for a healthy meal, a helpful strategy may be to always keep a healthy snack on hand (for example a bag of oil-free chips and a small container of salsa). This will, at the least, carry you over until you can find time or a place for a more substantial healthy meal. If, on the other hand, your cravings are associated with specific moods, emotions, or feelings, then assess if these can be better addressed without food or drink as a crutch. If not, then can you make healthier choices during these times of emotional eating/drinking? For instance, if you are longing for pizza, find a recipe for a healthier plant-based pizza (see Appendix I). Some possible recipe sources include drmcdougall.com, fatfreevegan.com, happycow.net, vegparadise.com, and pcrm.org (either look for their oil-free recipes or challenge yourself to substitute the oil in a recipe with healthy alternatives. See Appendix H). If you desire a hamburger and fries, get a veggie burger and oven-baked sweet potatoes. If you are craving chocolate cupcakes or carrot cake, check out Appendix I for some delicious recipes. The point is that these cravings will occur BUT that doesn't mean we have to satisfy them with unhealthy options. Instead, we can:

choose healthier versions,
as they exist for almost every craving.

We say "almost" because fortunately (or unfortunately for some of you) some yearnings cannot be substituted and therefore must simply be discontinued. For example, if you are craving a cigarette, although we could tell you to lick an ashtray, that would not be tempting, tasty, nor healthier.

Another important thing to remember is that these healthier versions will not be exact substitutions. Some won't taste quite the same, some will just taste different, but some will taste surprisingly better. That being said, taste is acquired and taste buds change over time. Have any of you switched from whole milk to skim milk or from regular cookies to their non-fat versions? If so, most of you will remember that initial "funny" change in taste. Over time you got used to the non-fat version, and if you ever went back to trying the regular version, then suddenly it tasted "funny." The same applies to these new food choices you will be making. So, have patience and maintain an open mind. The key here is to remember that we don't like everything we eat; it happens whether we are on a plant-based diet or not. So, if you are finding that your first few cooking attempts are not as tasty as you hoped, don't give up. Practice makes perfect, and this is no exception. There are so many options available to you on a plant-based diet, so just keep searching for new recipes and continue to experiment. Toss out the recipes you don't care for and hold on to the ones you like. Before you know it, you will have collected a repertoire of favorites (Thai peanut noodles, macaroni and "cheese," enchiladas, veggie burgers, sweet potato fries, split pea soup, tomato & basil pizza, chocolate muffins with peanut butter frosting) you and your family can enjoy again and again.

At this point, some of you are gung ho and ready to go. You may have already been contemplating a plant-based diet, or you find the benefits motivation enough to get started. By all means, begin right away - the sooner you transition, the sooner you begin to reap the benefits. But some of you may be feeling unsure. You may be concerned about a plant-based diet lacking protein, calcium, or vitamin B12. You may be challenging our claim that certain oils aren't health foods. And, you may not be convinced of all the benefits of converting to a plant-based diet. We hope that the next few chapters will help to dispel widespread myths, address common concerns, and answer your remaining questions.

Take-home messages:

- Our program revolves around two key findings:
  - There are no health benefits to eating animal foods over plant foods.
  - People are healthier on an oil-free, whole foods, plant-based diet.
- Aim to live in the "A" range of the Food Continuum[34]. If that is not possible, then do your best, remembering that doing a little (like adding one healthy dish per day) is better than doing nothing at all.
- The more natural whole foods you incorporate, the higher up you will move along the Food Continuum[34] as well as the Optimum Health Continuum.
- Follow the 3-Phase Eating Plan.
  - First course – your "weight loss medicine and multivitamin"
    - Vegetables (or fruit for breakfast)
  - Second course – your "filler"
    - Brown rice, potatoes, corn, oats, quinoa, bulgur, squash, legumes, etc.
  - Third course is optional
    - Whole-grain breads or pastas, corn tortillas, whole-grain chips or crackers, non-dairy milks, lasagna, pizza, burritos/enchiladas, etc.
- Monitor your deprivation.
- Address your cravings. (Remember that a healthier version exists for almost every craving, so challenge yourself to find and make it!)

Chapter 8: Protein

We begin with protein because, from our experience, most people who hear about a plant-based diet want to know, "Where would I get my protein?"

Let us begin with the basics. Proteins are composed of 20 amino acids, only 8 of which are essential, meaning that these have to be obtained from our food. It is a myth that only animal products provide enough of these essential amino acids. Another myth is that animal protein (believed to be the only source for complete proteins, containing all amino acids) is superior to plant protein. This notion was popularized by Frances Moore Lappe's original book *Diet for a Small Planet.* Lappe based her initial theory on studies done in the 1900s on rats. Based on these studies, she introduced the concept of "protein-combining" in which she recommended that people on a plant-based diet combine certain foods (like rice and beans) in order to form a "complete protein." Lappe has since recanted her belief in a revised version of her book (10 years later), now recognizing, along with most health experts, that protein combining is indeed unnecessary and that plant proteins *are* complete and *do* provide us with all of our essential amino acids. [35]

Studies on the effect of plant proteins on humans were, in fact, conducted as early as 1942 by Dr. William Rose, of the University of Illinois. His experiment involved testing his subjects by providing them with differing amounts of each of the eight essential amino acids (remember that these are the only amino acids our bodies cannot make on their own). He noted that after two days of receiving inadequate amounts of an essential amino acid, his subjects would inevitably begin to complain of nervousness, irritability, fatigue, and lack of appetite. They would also quickly go into negative nitrogen balance (indicating that more nitrogen, commonly found in protein, was being excreted than was being taken in).[36,37] With these observations, he was able to deduce the minimal intake requirement for each of these eight essential amino acids. He then recorded the highest level of need of a given essential amino acid and doubled it to

Keep it Simple, Keep it Whole

Table 2 – Essential Amino Acids in Various Foods compared to Rose's Minimum and Recommended Requirements

(grams per day) Amino Acids	Rose's Minimum Requirem.	Rose's Recomm. Requirem.	Corn	Brown Rice	Oatmeal Flakes	Wheat Flour	White Beans	Potatoes	Sweet Potatoes	Taro	Asparagus	Broccoli	Tomatoes	Pumpkin	Beef Club Steak	Egg	Milk
Tryptophan	.25	.50	.66	.71	1.4	1.4	1.8	.8	.8	1.0	3.9	3.8	1.4	1.5	3.1	3.8	2.3
Phenylalanine*	.28	.56	6.13	3.1	5.8	5.9	10.9	3.6	2.5	3.0	10.2	12.2	4.3	3.0	11.2	13.9	7.7
Leucine	1.10	2.20	12.0	5.5	8.1	8.0	17.0	4.1	2.6	5.2	14.6	16.5	6.1	6.0	22.4	21.0	15.9
Isoleucine	.7	1.4	4.1	3.0	5.6	5.2	11.3	3.6	2.2	3.0	11.9	12.8	4.4	4.3	14.3	15.7	10.3
Lysine	.8	1.6	4.1	2.5	4.0	3.2	14.7	4.4	2.1	3.4	15.5	14.8	6.3	5.5	23.9	15.3	12.5
Valine	.8	1.6	6.8	4.5	6.4	5.5	12.1	4.4	3.4	3.5	16.0	17.3	4.2	4.3	15.1	17.7	11.7
Methionine	.11	.22	2.1	1.1	1.6	1.8	2.0	1.0	.8	.6	5.0	5.1	1.1	1.0	6.8	7.4	3.9
Threonine	.5	1.0	4.5	2.5	3.6	3.5	8.5	3.4	2.1	2.7	9.9	12.5	4.9	2.7	12.1	12.0	7.4
Total Protein	20	37 (WHO)	109	64	108	120	198	82	45	58	330	338	150	115	276	238	160

Data gathered and compiled by John McDougall, MD

create a "definitely safe intake."[38] When Rose's minimum requirements are used to analyze a wide variety of plant foods, each of these foods is found to be in excess not only of his minimum requirement but also of his "definitely safe intake" (twice the minimum requirement) (see Table 2). So, as you can see,

> if we meet our daily caloric needs we would
> consume the essential amino acids in more
> than sufficient amounts, even if we were
> only eating one particular food.

To clarify, if you were only allowed to consume 500 calories a day, you would have a better chance of getting enough of all eight essential amino acids by consuming animal foods over plant foods (because per calorie animal products have more protein as well as more fat, cholesterol, and environmental toxins.) But, if you were only consuming 500 calories a day, you would be starving. In this case, getting enough essential amino acids would be the least of your worries, with the greater concern being getting enough calories to survive! Stated another way, you will only be protein-deficient if you are starving—and we could probably place a safe bet that most of you are not starving.

> The take-home message, then,
> is that as long as you are getting
> enough calories from nutritious, whole foods,
> meeting your protein requirement
> should no longer EVER concern you.

But that is easier said than done in a society where getting enough protein ranks up there with eating, breathing, and sleeping. This then begs the question, "How much protein do we actually need?"

> Since 1974, the World Health Organization
> has recommended that we get
> 5% of our calories from protein
> (6% during pregnancy).[39]

And this suggestion already incorporates a wide safety margin. To put things in perspective, human breast milk is 5% protein and is consumed by a baby who is doubling in size while only consuming that food. When was the last time we, as adults, needed to double in size? Why then, should the percentage of protein we, as adults, need be any greater (such as in the typical Western Diet, containing 10-35% protein)? How does 5% convert into our daily dietary needs, you may be wondering?

Well, proteins have 4 calories per gram. That means if you are a male requiring 3000 calories a day, your protein requirement is 38 grams (see Example 1).

Example 1: Calculating 5% protein for a male consuming 3000 calories/day.

Step 1 – Calculate 5% of 3000, which will give you the number of calories of protein that you need in one day.

$$3000 \text{ calories X .05 (or 5\%)} = 150 \text{ calories}$$

Step 2 – Calculate how many grams are in 150 calories (remember that for every gram there are 4 calories of protein).

$$150 \text{ calories x } \frac{1 \text{ gram}}{4 \text{ calories}} = 37.5 \text{ g (about 38 grams)}$$

Step 3 – Conclusion

A male eating 3000 calories per day requires about 38 grams of protein (the weight of about 8 nickels).

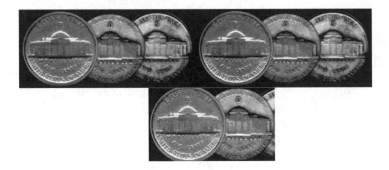

If you are a woman burning 2300 calories a day, then you require 29 grams of protein (see Example 2).

Example 2: Calculating 5% protein for a woman consuming 2300 calories/day.

Step 1 – Calculate 5% of 2300, which will give you the number of calories of protein that you need in one day.

$$2300 \text{ calories X } .05 \text{ (or } 5\%) = 115 \text{ calories}$$

Step 2 – Calculate how many grams are in 115 calories (remember that for every gram there are 4 calories of protein).

$$115 \text{ calories x } \frac{1 \text{ gram}}{4 \text{ calories}} = 28.75 \text{ g (about 29 grams)}$$

Step 3 – Conclusion

A woman eating 2300 calories per day
requires about 29 grams of protein
(the weight of about 6 nickels).

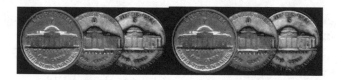

To get an idea of the weight of a gram, 1 gram = 0.035 ounces (16 ounces = 1 pound) and a U.S. nickel weighs about 5 grams. So, 38 grams (daily protein recommendation for a male) would be the weight of about 8 nickels and 29 grams (daily protein recommendation for a female) would be the weight of about 6 nickels (see Examples 1 and 2 above).

How do we meet this requirement? Contrary to popular belief, this is not a difficult feat. Brown rice is 9% protein, potatoes are 10% protein, wheat flour is 18% protein, oatmeal is 19% protein, black beans are 35% protein, mushrooms are 35% protein, asparagus is 43% protein, and the list goes on and on.

Table 3 - Percent Calories from Protein in Various Foods

Food	Percent Calories from Protein (%)
Brown Rice	9%
Potatoes	10%
Wheat Flour	18%
Oatmeal	19%
Black Beans	35%
Mushrooms	35%
Asparagus	43%

J Pennington. Bowes and Church's Food Values of Portions Commonly Used.
17th Ed. Lippincott. Philadelphia-New York. 1998.

The point is that you can easily meet your protein requirement on a plant-based diet. For example, 2000 calories of oats has 87 grams of protein and far exceeds the minimum requirement for all 8 essential amino acids. Again, the only exception to this is if you are not meeting your daily caloric requirements with primarily nutritious whole foods (vegetables, fruits, whole grains, legumes, etc.)

So for all the carnivores out there convinced that animal products are the only source of protein, wake up and taste the broccoli!

Broccoli has a higher percentage of protein than pork, salmon, chicken, skim milk, eggs, beef, and cheddar cheese![40]
(see Table 4)

Table 4 - Percent Calories from Protein Various Foods Compared to Broccoli

Food	Percent Calories from Protein (%)
Broccoli	50%
Pork	45%
Salmon	44%
Chicken	42%
Skim Milk	40%
Eggs	35%
Beef	34%
Cheddar Cheese	25%

J Pennington. Bowes and Church's Food Values of Portions Commonly Used.
17th Ed. Lippincott. Philadelphia-New York. 1998.

And more importantly, the broccoli does not come with the laundry list of problems associated with animal products.

What is this laundry list? Let us begin with the fact that,

animal based diets provide excessive amounts of protein.

Although that may sound like a great thing to some of you, in actuality, "too much of a good thing" can indeed be harmful. The reality is that our liver and kidneys filter out excess protein. When we consume protein in excess, it stresses the kidneys to work harder. Eventually, their function deteriorates. You may not realize this is happening because the human body can compensate exceptionally well. We know that a 50% loss of kidney function is not a problem as people can live a full, healthy life with only one kidney. As a matter of fact, you need to lose a significant amount of your kidney function before it becomes really noticeable.[41]

Furthermore, proteins are composed of amino ACIDS and are therefore acidic by nature. The problem here is that our bodies function best when they are in a slightly alkaline or basic state (in other words, the opposite of acidic).

Proteins are acidic by nature BUT
our bodies function best in a slightly basic state
(i.e., just the opposite environment).

When we eat too many proteins, we introduce too much acidity into the body. One way to neutralize this acidity is by eating fruits and vegetables, which are, by nature, mostly alkaline (basic). Another way, and much more common in the Western Diet of high protein and few fruits and vegetables, is for our bones to release calcium and other such buffers to neutralize the acid. Over time, this loss of calcium weakens the bones and may lead to problems like osteoporosis. In fact, a National Institute of Health study at the University of California, published in the American Journal of Clinical Nutrition (2001), found that "women who ate most of their protein from animal sources had three times the rate of bone loss and 3.7 times the rate of hip fractures as women who ate most of their protein from vegetable sources."[42]

Another problem with animal products is that
they are very high in calories.

Compare 100 grams of beef (282 calories) or chicken (246 calories) to 100 grams of brown rice (110 calories), potatoes (100 calories), bananas (90 calories), apples (59 calories), or broccoli (28 calories).

Table 5 - Calories in 100g of Various Foods

Food	Calories in 100 grams
Beef	282
Chicken	246
Brown Rice	110
Potatoes	100
Banana	90
Apples	59
Broccoli	28

J Pennington. Bowes and Church's Food Values of Portions Commonly Used.
17th Ed. Lippincott. Philadelphia-New York. 1998.

Animal products are also very high in fat.

Again, compare beef (as high as 66% fat), chicken (58%), or pork (55%) to broccoli (15%), brown rice (7%), apples (6%,) bananas (4%), or potatoes (1%).

The combination of high levels of calories and high amounts of fat is not only disastrous to our weight but also to our general health.
Here's why:

Our hunger/satiation signals are much less sensitive to fat.

Table 6 - Percent Calories from Fat in Various Foods

Food	Percent Calories from Fat (%)
Beef	66%
Chicken	58%
Pork	55%
Broccoli	15%
Brown Rice	7%
Apples	6%
Bananas	4%
Potatoes	1%

J Pennington. Bowes and Church's Food Values of Portions Commonly Used.
17th Ed. Lippincott. Philadelphia-New York. 1998.

One hypothesis to explain this is that satiation is signaled by caloric density through primarily stretch of our stomachs. In plain English, that means that our stomachs respond to the volume of food that we eat as well as the calories we are consuming, what we like to call our "calorie currency." Just as the beating of our heart and the expansion of our lungs occur automatically, so does the signal to the body as to how many calories it needs in a day. When we eat a whole foods and mostly plant-based diet, as did our ancestors, this feedback system works extremely competently. The reason for this is that these

whole foods have a good ratio of calories to bulk (water and fiber); they are the "calorie currency" our body evolved on.

For example, 3000 calories of fruits and vegetables have over 100 grams of fiber and over 5 liters of water. This mechanism does not work nearly as well when we eat high-fat, calorie-dense animal products and processed foods, which have a high number of calories despite being a much smaller volume of food. In this case, we send mixed messages to our bodies, resulting in confusion and inefficiency.

Let us use an example to clarify. A large fast food hamburger (32.8 grams of fat or 51% of total calories from fat), medium French fries (18.9 grams of fat or 46% total calories from fat), and 20oz. soda together equal about 1120 calories (51 grams of fat or 41% total calories from fat – the total percent of fat decreased, as the soda has calories but no fat). Compare that to 6 ½ medium-sized baked potatoes with salsa at 1100 calories (1 gram of fat or 1% total calories from fat).

Figure 7 - Comparing Calories and Fat: A Fast Food Meal versus Baked Potatoes

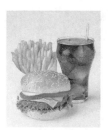 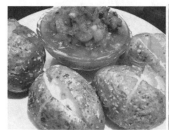

Total Calories: 1120
Total Fat: 51 grams
(41% fat calories)

Total Calories: 1100
Total Fat: 1 gram
(1% fat calories)

Which one do you think will fill you up more? If you answered the hamburger then you have never tried to eat that many baked potatoes! The sheer volume of the potatoes and the stretch that they create in your stomach will signal to your brain that you are full (and satiated) much more rapidly than the volume and stretch created by the fast food meal. Thinking of it another way, the average American male (35-50 years old, 5 feet 10 inches, weighing about 190 pounds, and lightly active) requires about 2400 calories a day; whereas the average

American female (35-50 years old, 5 foot 4 inches, weighing 140 pounds, and lightly active) requires about 1700 calories a day. Dividing this by three for breakfast, lunch, and dinner (so this does NOT include snacks) comes out to about 800 calories per meal for a male and about 560 calories per meal for a female. Applying our knowledge from the above paragraph, our stomach estimates how much stretch it needs to fulfill that calorie requirement (800 for a male and 560 for a female). Eating the medium-sized baked potatoes (4 ½ for a male and 3 for a female) (see Figure 8) delivers the adequate volume as well as the appropriate number of calories. Our stretched stomach is now satisfied that it received enough energy (or calories) from this meal and signals to our brain that it is full. Now, let us apply this same model to the fast food meal. To remain within the caloric requirement, a male would only be able to eat about two-thirds of his hamburger and French fries and half of his soda; while a female would only be able to eat half of her hamburger, fries, and soda (see Figure 8).

Figure 8 – Amount of Food That Can Be Eaten to Meet the Average Calorie Requirement of a Typical Meal for a Male and a Female.

For a male:

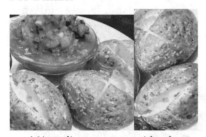 vs.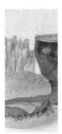

4 ½ medium potatoes with salsa   2/3 hamburger, 2/3 fries, ½ soda

For a female:

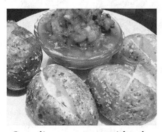 vs.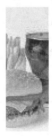

3 medium potatoes with salsa   ½ hamburger, ½ fries, ½ soda

The reduction in this meal results in less volume and therefore less stretch. Our stomach becomes confused because it is not adequately stretched and therefore believes it has not consumed enough calories. It then sends the signal to our body that we must eat more to meet our caloric requirement. So, we finish our burger, fries, and soda, at which point we have over-consumed by about 320 calories for a male and 560 calories for a female. If we continue to overshoot by this many calories per meal for only ONE of our three meals a day, an average male will gain about 3 pounds a month (that's 36 pounds a year!) and an average female will gain about 5 pounds a month (that's 60 pounds a year!). Not to mention that by doing so, we fail to get the essential vitamins, minerals, and phytochemicals that are found primarily in plant-based foods.

This is a really important concept so let us use one more example to make sure we have made our point. A regular sized chocolate candy bar (2oz) is about 270 calories, with the king size being (4 oz) about 540 calories. Compare that to a medium-sized apple at about 90 calories and a large apple at about 115 calories. You can have 3 medium sized apples (270 calories) for every one regular-sized candy bar or about 4.5 large apples (520 calories) for every king-sized candy bar. Choosing the apples will give your body not only the stretch and the calories in the appropriate amounts it requires, but it will also provide you with the vitamins, minerals, phytochemicals, and fiber that your body needs to function optimally. And, it will do this without loading you up with unhealthy and damaging calories from fat.

> Remember that animal products and processed foods are deficient and often devoid of vitamins, minerals, fiber, water, and phytochemicals.

Okay, so you get the volume and calorie deal. But are we saying that you have to eat only potatoes and apples? Hardly! In fact, your food choices on a low-fat, plant-based diet are not only endless, they are simultaneously satisfying and delicious (see recipes in Appendix I for some ideas). This exercise was only intended to demonstrate how easy it is for us to over-consume when we eat processed, fatty foods.

The over-consumption then cascades into a myriad of other health issues. To begin with, these excess calories get stored as fat in our bellies, hips, butts, and thighs. But obesity is not the only health problem associated with excess fat consumption. Fat in our bodies also promotes the production of estrogen, and excess estrogen has been linked to precocious puberty, fibroids, and uterine and breast cancer.[43] In addition,

the fat we find in most animal products
is devoid of essential fats (omega-3 and omega-6, both
produced only by plants) and is mostly saturated fat.

This saturated fat raises our cholesterol, clogs our arteries, and increases our risk for heart disease (the number one killer in the United States). Finally, fat that can build up inside cells, known as intramyocellular lipid, is thought to be a major factor in the inhibition of the action of insulin on the cells in the body.[44] When insulin is not working properly, it cannot guide glucose (sugar) into our cells. The glucose then stays in the bloodstream and raises our blood sugars, damaging our eyes, kidneys, nerves, and blood vessels and causing the growing health problem better known as diabetes.

Notice that we didn't differentiate between chicken, turkey, pork, and beef. Many studies have focused on meat, concluding that total meat consumption is directly linked to cancer of the stomach, colon, rectum, pancreas, lung, breast, prostate, testis, kidney, and bladder.[45] In addition meat, especially when processed, has been shown to increase overall risk of death as well as death from cancer and heart disease.[46] But, although red meat has taken the flak as a convenient scapegoat for all the "badness" associated with animal products, the reality is that, as Dr. John McDougall likes to say,

"a muscle is a muscle is a muscle"

regardless of what form it comes in, and is therefore equally hazardous to your health. All of these animal products are high in protein (chicken 42%, turkey 52%, pork 45%, beef 34%), high in fat (chicken 58%, turkey 48%, pork 55%, and beef 66%), and high in cholesterol (in 100 grams of: chicken 91mg, turkey 89mg, pork 84mg, beef 90mg). It is worthwhile to note here that all plant foods have zero cholesterol.

Table 7 – Comparing Calories from Protein, Fat and Cholesterol in Chicken, Turkey, Pork, and Beef

Food	Percent Calories from Protein (%)	Percent Calories from Fat (%)	Cholesterol (mg/100g of food)
Chicken	42%	58%	91mg
Turkey	52%	48%	89mg
Pork	45%	55%	84mg
Beef	34%	66%	90mg

J Pennington. Bowes and Church's Food Values of Portions Commonly Used.
17th Ed. Lippincott. Philadelphia-New York. 1998.

Note that these numbers are averages, and although we can modify them, that does not necessarily make them healthier. For example, we can remove the fat from chicken but then we just increase its protein content. Knowing what we already know about excess proteins, this is like choosing cancer over heart disease. Putting data like this together, with other epidemiological evidence supporting the many benefits of a plant-based diet (such as *The China Study*, written by nutrition expert and health researcher T. Colin Campbell, PhD.), we can see that

all animal products are equally responsible for contributing to obesity, cancer, heart disease, and diabetes.

For those of you who have eliminated land animals and have moved onto sea animals, stay tuned, this section is for you.

Remember that "a muscle is a muscle is a muscle," and fish are no exception.

In fact, fish have just as much cholesterol as beef, chicken, or pork (mg/100grams: chicken 91, beef 90, pork 84, salmon 64, halibut 59, tuna 58).

Table 8 – Amount of Cholesterol (mg) in 100 grams of Various Foods

Food	Cholesterol (mg/100g of food)
Chicken	91mg
Beef	90mg
Pork	84mg
Salmon	64mg
Halibut	59mg
Tuna	58mg

J Pennington. Bowes and Church's Food Values of Portions Commonly Used.
17th Ed. Lippincott. Philadelphia-New York. 1998.

An increase in fish intake has also been associated with an increase in breast cancer. In a study published in the Journal of Nutrition, researchers found that "For each 25 grams (less than one ounce) of lean fish consumed daily there was a 13% increase in risk of breast cancer. For fatty fish the increase was 11% for each 25 grams."[47]

Fish are also laden with contaminants. Of particular concern in recent years are mercury and PCBs (polychlorinated biphenyls – industrial compounds banned in the U.S. in 1976 but persist because of their widespread use and their ability to linger in the environment).[48] Contamination with these toxins has been linked to increased risks of heart attacks, cancer, increased total and LDL ("bad") cholesterol, suppression of the immune system, memory loss, learning disabilities, and depression. [49,50, 51, 52] But fish are rich in omega-3 so doesn't that make them a health food? No! As a matter of fact, fish today are so contaminated with environmental pollutants, such as mercury, that these toxins have been found to neutralize any theoretical benefits of the omega-3 content.[53] And, contrary to popular belief, fish do not create omega-3 fats; they get them from the plants they eat (see more about this in chapter 11, Fats and Oils). Why, then, shouldn't we do the same, especially if that means we can avoid the high cholesterol and chemical toxicity?

You might be asking yourself at this point, if the ocean is polluted with these chemicals, don't the plants take them up as well? Great question. The answer is yes; unfortunately the plants will absorb some of those chemicals. BUT, and this is a big but, they absorb them in much smaller amounts than do the fish. The reason for this is twofold: first, plants are low in fat, and these chemicals are lipophilic (meaning they like to hide in fat). Second, plants are low on the food chain while animals are high on the food chain. Through a process known as bio-magnification, the higher up on the food chain something is, the more toxicity it carries.

Looking at Figure 9, we can see that a plant may absorb, let's say, 5 units (parts per million) of these chemicals. Fish eat many plants, and for EACH one they eat, they get 5 units; this is the process of magnification. The fish then store these contaminants in their body. By the time we eat the fish, they have accumulated a large amount of these toxic contaminants. We, like the animals, also store these toxins in our bodies. The only way to get rid of them is by eliminating them from our diet and allowing them to break down over time. For example, dioxin one of the most carcinogenic environmental toxins that exists, has a half-life of 7 years. In other words, if we had 100 fgs (femtograms) of dioxin in our bodies today and did not consume anymore of it, then in 7 years we would bring that level down to 50 fgs and in another 7 years (14 years later) we would be down to 25 fgs, and so on. It is worthwhile to note that the Environmental Protection Agency says that 93% of our dioxin exposure comes from consuming animal products, in particular fish and dairy.[54]

Not only does that wreak havoc in our systems but we then pass it on to our children. In fact, according to the U.S. Environmental Protection Agency, nursing infants can absorb up to 90-100% of the PCBs present in breast milk.[55] They further state that "breast-fed infants may have an increased risk because of the bio-concentration of PCBs in breast milk," and that embryos, fetuses, and neonates may be particularly susceptible to PCB toxicity, as their underdevelopment may make it easier for them to accumulate these contaminants.[56] Some of the health effects seen with babies born to mothers who have been exposed to high levels of PCBs include: lower birth weight, smaller head circumference, impaired short-term memory, and slower responsiveness.[57] It is no wonder that the U.S. Defense Fund told women eating fish not to breast feed back in the 1970s! Even then, they were aware of the health hazards of the "chicken" of the sea.

Figure 9 – Bio-Magnification in the Food Chain

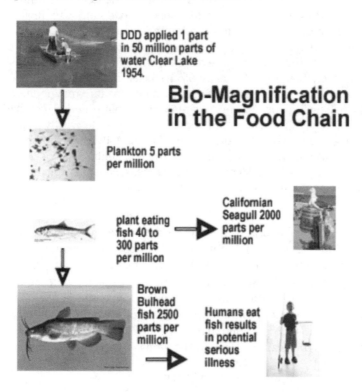

Hopefully at this stage, if we have done nothing more, we have convinced you that you can meet your daily protein requirement by eating only plants. But what about iron? Don't animals provide more iron than plants? Isn't iron from animal sources more readily absorbed? Aren't most vegetarians and vegans iron-deficient? Like omega fatty acids (previously discussed), animals do not make iron;

iron is a mineral that comes from the ground and is absorbed by plants.

Animals obtain iron by eating the plants.

Although many people worry about not getting enough iron, the reality is that most cases of iron-deficiency are not a result of insufficient iron intake. Rather, they are the result of blood loss secondary to internal bleeding (ulcers, inflammatory bowel disease, uterine fibroids, etc.), use of certain medications (NSAIDs such as aspirin and ibuprofen), heavy menstrual cycles, and cancer, among other things. In fact, most people eating the typical American diet will actually have an iron surplus. Over time, this excess iron accumulation wreaks havoc in the body. Symptoms of iron overload can be mild or severe depending on the extent of the overload and can include fatigue, weakness, painful joints, abdominal pain, vascular damage, darkening of the skin, frequent urination, and increased risk of infections.[58,59] Ultimately, iron overload can lead to liver disease (enlarged liver, scarring of the liver/cirrhosis, liver failure, and/or liver cancer), heart disease (irregular heart beats and/or heart failure), diabetes, arthritis, chronic abdominal pain, and decreased thyroid function.[60] Iron reduction, especially in people with vascular disease (arguably most older Americans), has actually been shown not only to decrease the risk of getting cancer by 35% but also to decrease overall mortality by 51%![61] The take-home message is that for most of us, getting enough iron should not be a concern.

As for the absorption question, nature has developed the perfect solution for both plants and animals to maximize their iron intake. Plant iron (non-heme iron) is not as readily absorbed as animal iron (heme iron), and that is possibly a protective feature (as more iron is not necessarily better). But, to compensate for this fact, plants (unlike animals) are loaded with vitamin C, which helps to regulate and increase iron absorption. In addition, plant foods often contain more iron than animal sources. Compare how much iron (in milligrams or mg) is found in 100 grams of each of the foods in Table 9.

Once again, the take-home message is that,

a plant-based diet rich in fruits, vegetables, whole grains, and legumes will provide you with sufficient amounts of iron, without exposing you to all of the health hazards associated with eating animal products.

Table 9 – Amount of Iron (mg) in 100 grams of Various Foods

Food	Iron (mg/100g of food)
pumpkin and squash seed kernels	15.1mg
white beans cooked	3.7mg
lentils cooked	3.3mg
spinach cooked	3.2mg
shrimp	3.1mg
beef	2.4mg
prime rib	2.3mg
roasted chicken	1.4mg
pork	1.1mg
salmon	.34mg

J Pennington. Bowes and Church's Food Values of Portions Commonly Used. 17th Ed. Lippincott. Philadelphia-New York. 1998.

Okay, so no animals, but what about dairy? Isn't milk good for our body and bones? Again, that would be an emphatic NO, but we will discuss dairy in Chapter 10. For those of you aiming this book at the trash can, remember that we are not telling you never to eat animal products. We are not asking you to cancel next weekend's barbeque. And we are not expecting you to give up your sushi or your fish tacos. What we are saying is that animal products pose hazards to your health. They increase your risk for many serious and fatal diseases, including our top killers: heart disease and cancer. Furthermore, they lead to obesity and other chronic diseases, such as diabetes, high blood pressure, and osteoporosis. These are the foods that rate a D or an F on the Food Continuum[34]. They are also the food choices that move the "Diet" portion, the "Disease Elimination" portion (because they increase risk of disease), and the "Off Pills" portion (because they increase the likelihood you will require prescriptions) of your Optimum Health Continuum (OHC) in the wrong direction (i.e., to the left when our goal is to get you to the right). Our objective is simply to deliver the science, the facts that will help you make more informed decisions as you choose whether or not to incorporate these foods into your diet.

Take-home messages:

- Plant proteins are NOT inferior to animal proteins, AND they provide us with all of the essential amino acids.

- The World Health Organization recommends we get 5% of our calories from protein (6% during pregnancy).

- The typical Western diet contains 10-35% protein.

- You are getting more than enough protein as long as you are meeting your caloric need with nutritious foods.

- A plant-based diet of fruits, vegetables, whole grains, and legumes will provide you with sufficient amounts of iron.

- Problems with animal products:

  o High in protein (stresses the liver and kidneys and may lead to osteoporosis

  o High in calories (leads to obesity and obesity-related diseases)

  o High in fat (leads to clogging of the arteries, high cholesterol, heart disease, and diabetes)

  o Lack vitamins, minerals, essential fats, phytochemicals, fiber essential for optimum health)

- Our hunger/satiation signals are much less sensitive to dietary fat (found in significant amounts in animal products), so it is very easy for us to over-consume when eating these foods.

- "A muscle is a muscle is a muscle": chicken, turkey, beef, pork, and fish are equally hazardous to our health.

- Fish has just as much cholesterol as beef, chicken, or pork and is laden with environmental contaminants).

- All animal products equally contribute to obesity, cancer, heart disease, and diabetes.

Chapter 9: Soy

In the last chapter we discussed the fact that you could meet your protein requirement with whole plant foods alone. Although that leaves us with a lot of choices, many people focus on soy and soy products. Maybe this is because so many animal product substitutes are made from soy derivatives. Things like soy chicken, soy burgers, soy taco mix, soy cheese, etc., are rampant in our markets. Or maybe it is because advertisements everywhere are touting the benefits of soy. But what is the real story with soy? The truth is that the jury is still out.

For example, isoflavones in soy mimic estrogen, and increased estrogen in the body may promote the growth of estrogen-sensitive cancers. However, studies have shown that isoflavones from soy can inhibit prostate and breast cancer and that these cancers have a decreased incidence in countries like China and Japan (where soy products are consumed regularly).[62] One study looked at genistein levels in the blood (an isoflavone that correlates with soy intake) and noted over a 50% reduction in initial occurrence of breast cancer in people with higher levels of genistein.[63] Another study in women who already had estrogen-receptor-positive breast cancer showed that those with the highest levels of isoflavones (commonly found in soy) in their blood actually reduced their all-cause mortality by nearly half! In other words, they were less likely to die if they had higher levels of isoflavones in their blood. They hypothesized that soy phytoestrogens, which are less stimulating, bind to estrogen receptors in the breast and block the more stimulating ovarian estrogen.[64] This doesn't mean you should or should not eat soy, as many plant foods contain these substances, but it also makes a good case that soy is not necessarily an evil food.

Another controversial topic is heart disease. Some studies show that soy products can lower cholesterol and, therefore, decrease risk of heart disease, while others show there is minimal to no heart benefit.[65,66,67]

Soy's effects on the immune system are also on the fence. While some studies show that soy isoflavones suppress the immune system others suggest that they boost immune function.[68,69] Studies on soy's effect on thyroid function have met similar ambiguity. On one hand, studies have associated autoimmune thyroid disorder with soy consumption as well as linked goiter and hypothyroidism to infant soy formulas.[70] On the other hand, studies have shown that soy may be protective against thyroid disorders, particularly thyroid cancer.[71]

Although the message regarding soy is confusing and the debate continues, it is important to note that this controversy extends only to natural soy products (e.g., edamame, tofu, tempeh, miso).

There is no confusion about processed soy products, as they are clearly NOT health foods.

Processed soy products include soy presented as hydrolyzed soy protein, isolated soy protein, soy or soy protein concentrates, textured vegetable protein, soy lecithin, and soybean oil. These synthetically manufactured products can be just as harmful as animal products. They often are: genetically manipulated (modification of food has been associated with organ damage, immune system impairment, and higher risk of causing allergic reactions and autoimmune responses), high in protein (which leads to destruction of kidney function as well as osteoporosis), and have been found to significantly increase insulin-like growth factor-1 (a protein responsible for cell growth as well as promoting cancer and accelerating aging).[72,73] Hopefully these are reasons enough to convince you to eliminate, or at least minimize, the amount of processed soy products you consume.

As for the other "natural" soy products like tofu, tempeh, edamame, soy sauce (as a general note, stick to Tamari or Shoyu, as these tend to use organic soybeans and do not contain MSG or artificial favoring/coloring), and miso, many studies demonstrating the benefits of soy do so by studying Asian populations, particularly in China and Japan. If we are choosing to include soy products in our diet, why not follow their example? To do so, we should start by finding out how much soy is really incorporated in the Asian diets. According to a study published in the Journal of Nutrition,

"The average daily consumption of soy, in Japan, was about 63 grams for men and 54 grams for women."[74] This translates into a little over a quarter of a cup!

Data from China is roughly the same, with average daily soy protein consumption at about 60 grams for men and about 70 grams for women.[75] The take-home message here is that these are very small quantities of soy, used mostly to flavor foods and not as the main course. This is in great contrast to our tofu dishes with a few vegetables or our tempeh loaf and small salad.

Ultimately, there is no one miracle or "magic-bullet" food, and soy is no exception.

This is, unfortunately, the reductionist "quick-fix" theory that gets us into trouble again and again. We learn about a product, in this case soy, which is after all just a bean (but you can easily substitute olive oil, supplements, etc., here as well), take the information completely out of context and then expect to get astounding benefits. What is happening here is that we are failing to look at the big picture in which **no** one food is a "cure-all." For example, studies consistently report that people eating soy generally have healthier diets (higher in whole plant foods and lower in animal products and processed foods) than those not incorporating soy into their diets. The soy then is not necessarily the health tonic, rather it is most likely the soy in combination with the high amounts of plant foods and low amounts of animal/processed foods that produce the favorable results. It is for this reason that adding soy (in any form) to the disease-promoting American diet and lifestyle will not reverse disease.

Our best advice to you, if you choose to include soy products in your diet, is the following:

1) Use traditional forms (tofu, tempeh, miso, soymilk, tamari) over synthetically processed forms (burgers, cheese, hot dogs, protein bars, etc.).
2) Even when you use traditional forms of soy, use them in moderation as condiments or flavorings for your food and not as the main course (remember that soy is a richer and higher fat food).
3) If you must have the synthetic, processed soy products, make this an exception, and consume them on rare occasions.
4) Remember that there is no need to add soy to a plant-based diet to get enough protein.

Take-home messages:

- You can meet your protein requirement with whole plant foods alone.

- Processed soy products are NOT health foods.

- The benefits of soy have been demonstrated through studies of populations consuming traditional soy products in very small amounts.

- There is no one miracle or "magic-bullet" food.

- Adding soy (in any form) to the disease-promoting American diet and lifestyle will NOT reverse disease.

  o When using soy be sure to use the traditional forms and do so in moderation.

Chapter 10: Dairy

Second to protein, our next biggest hurdle has been teaching people that they can get sufficient amounts of calcium on a plant-based diet. If you think about it, where does calcium come from?

Calcium is a mineral found in the earth.
Plants absorb calcium (and all minerals)
through their roots. Animals, eating these calcium-rich
plants, are then able to absorb the mineral
and store it in their bones.

Sound familiar? (See discussion on iron in Chapter 8.) The same would happen to us if we went directly to the source. Just look at all the other herbivores out there, including horses, cows, giraffes, rhinos, and elephants. These animals have large skeletons and strong bones and all from eating only plant foods. The take-home message here is, if they can sustain their large frames on a plant-based diet, we should have no problem sustaining ours.

The irony is that for all of our concern, there has never been a documented case of calcium deficiency in otherwise healthy people on natural diets.[76] In fact, most people eating the typical western diet consume more calcium than they likely need.

The average calcium intake in most Western countries
is about 800-1000mg/day.[77]

That is **one and a half to two times** the 500 milligrams per day recommended by the World Health Organization.[78]

So, why do we worry? We worry because we are bombarded by misinformation. Most of us are probably familiar with the slogans, "Milk, it does a body good" or "Got milk?" These advertisements are part of a multi-million-dollar campaign to promote dairy products as not only good for us but essential for our health and proper development. We have been duped into believing such erroneous claims as: consuming dairy is the only way to build strong bones or eating three servings of dairy a day will help you lose weight.

The reality about dairy is not nearly so glamorous. The Dairy Industry is forced to discuss calcium because that is the only mineral found in milk in any significant amount. And, despite that calcium, milk still does not give us the benefits the dairy industry boasts it does. In fact, numerous studies have shown that

populations that consume more dairy products are MORE prone to bone fractures.

Specifically, the Journal of Pediatrics reported that "in clinical, longitudinal, retrospective, and cross-sectional studies, neither increased consumption of dairy products, specifically, nor total dietary calcium consumption has shown even a modestly consistent benefit for child or young adult bone health."[79] Another study, a meta-analysis published in the British Medical Journal, looked at 19 studies assessing the effectiveness of calcium supplementation on bone mineral density. The study concluded that "calcium supplementation does not improve bone mineral density in children especially in the vertebral column and hips, (areas) which really matter as these are the sites of fractures in later life."[80] They also noted that:

long-term calcium supplementation comes with its own dangers,

in particular, increased calcium in the blood (hypercalcemia), which can cause symptoms from nausea and vomiting to weakness and muscle/joint pains to irregular heartbeats and coma. The study also concluded that calcium inhibits vitamin D conversion into its active form. The editorial following this meta-analysis added that, "Populations that consume the most cow's milk and other dairy products have among the highest rates of osteoporosis and hip fracture in later life."[81] This finding was supported by yet another study stating that "Consumption of dairy products, particularly at age 20 years, was associated with an increased risk of hip fractures" later in life.[82] Likewise, a Harvard Study of 78,000 women also came to the same conclusion. They reported that, "Data indicate that frequent milk consumption and higher dietary calcium intakes in middle-aged women do not provide protection against hip or forearm fractures. (Furthermore), women consuming greater amounts of calcium from dairy foods had significantly increased risks of hip fractures, while no increase in fracture risk was observed for the same levels of calcium from non-dairy sources."[83] Not convinced? Just look at population studies for further proof. Countries that consume the most milk, like the United States, Sweden, and England, have the highest rates of osteoporosis while countries that consume fewer dairy products, like Hong-Kong and Singapore, have much lower rates of osteoporosis.[84]

A large part of the problem is that,

> ## dairy products are high in protein, and "Osteoporosis is caused by a number of things, one of the most important being too much dietary protein."[85]

We have already learned that increased protein consumption introduces excess acid into our bodies, which respond by moving calcium out of our bones to neutralize this acid. "Even when eating 1,400mg of calcium a day, one can lose up to 4% of his or her bone mass each year on a high-protein diet."[86]

What about vitamin D? Many ask whether milk is a necessary source for vitamin D. Yet in reality,

> ## most of the vitamin D in milk is added to it.

In fact, unfortified milk has a very small amount of vitamin D - compare unfortified milk, which contains 0.3ug vitamin D (12 IU) to fortified milk, which contains 12ug vitamin D (480 IU).[87] Even with the supplemented vitamin D, 480 IU isn't going to provide nearly enough vitamin D for people to optimize their levels. Furthermore, vitamin D supplementation is not exclusive to milk. Other products such as juices, cereals, breads, and crackers are also fortified with vitamin D. But more importantly,

> ## vitamin D is a hormone that is naturally made in our skin upon exposure to sunlight.

In theory, with adequate exposure, over 90% of our vitamin D should come from sunlight. For most of us, that means exposing our arms, legs, torso, and face (ideally expose 50-75% of the skin surface) for a mere 15 minutes, three to four times a week. (For more information on sunlight exposure requirements, which takes into account UV index and skin tone, please read our website article about vitamin D, at: www.exsalus.com/Site/H_I_4_Vitamin_D.html.) In fact, with optimal exposure, most people can make up to 10,000 IU of vitamin D per day.[88] Note that after adequate time is spent (usually 15 minutes, depending on skin tone and UV index) and we have made the necessary amount of vitamin D for the day, our skin reaches an equilibrium and we don't make anymore vitamin D. In other words, unlike with supplements, we can't make ourselves toxic with vitamin D from sun exposure.

As for the claim that dairy makes you trim, that too, is just another myth. Just think of the original function of dairy, which is to help grow a 60lb calf into a 600lb cow. Why should we think it would perform any differently in our bodies? In fact, more and more studies show that an

increase in dairy product consumption results in weight gain NOT weight loss.

A review article funded by the dairy industry (yes, you read that correctly) took a look at nine studies correlating dairy intake with weight changes. Of these nine studies, seven showed that dairy consumption resulted in no change in weight and the other two studies showed weight GAIN when dairy was added.[89] These are studies funded by the dairy industry, made up of people who have a vested interest (both monetary and reputation) in making dairy products appear beneficial, yet the best they could do was come up with studies that showed no weight change with dairy consumption. That is, of course, the best-case scenario with dairy intake, because the other scenario is actual weight gain. Another study, published in the June 2005 Archives of Pediatrics & Adolescent Medicine, observed teenagers and dairy consumption. They found that teenagers drinking more than three glasses of milk a day actually gained, not lost, weight.[90] When you think of teenagers drinking one to two cartons of milk with each school meal, three glasses a day seems rather easy to consume. Let's look at one more study, a meta-analysis that looked at 49 clinical trials (from 1966 through 2007) evaluating the effects of dairy products or calcium intake on body weight. Their conclusion: "Evidence from the [49] trials showed that neither dairy products nor calcium supplements helped people lose weight."[91]

It is bad enough that dairy intake increases your risk for bone fractures and could result in weight gain, but as far as what is wrong with dairy, that is only the tip of the iceberg.

Dairy, in the simplest of terms, is liquid meat.

That being said, all of the negatives associated with eating meat are equally linked with eating dairy. This includes the increased calories, fat, protein, and cholesterol as well as the heart disease, diabetes, osteoporosis, and cancer. In addition, dairy is closely linked to chronic constipation, especially in children. A New England Journal of Medicine study showed that there was a 68% reduction in severe constipation in children when dairy was removed from their diet. Interestingly, when dairy was reintroduced a year later, ALL children redeveloped constipation within 5-10 days.[92]

For those of you thinking you are off the hook for drinking skim milk, read on. Skimming milk actually increases the protein and lactose content (this is because you remove the fat layer and leave the protein/lactose-rich layer).

An increase in protein (consisting of amino *acids*) causes our body to release material (specifically calcium, which is *basic*) from our bones to provide a neutralizing buffer.

This process eventually leads to osteoporosis. As for lactose, many people are unable to digest this milk sugar. Increasing the proportion of lactose in milk only leads to more diarrhea, cramps, and gas.

Dairy protein is also known to be a
major cause of food allergies.

Dairy is extremely mucous-producing for some people and can irritate and clog the entire respiratory system, resulting in allergies, asthma, sinusitis, colds, runny noses, and ear infections. See it with your own eyes when an infant or child eliminates dairy and their Eustachian tube inflammation, swelling, and resulting chronic ear infections magically resolve. Furthermore, dairy proteins have similar amino acid sequences to proteins in our pancreas. Our body responds to these proteins as foreign invaders and makes antibodies to mount an immune response against these milk proteins. The problem is that because the proteins on our pancreas look so similar, our body attacks them as well. The destruction of the pancreas then leads to type I diabetes. Studies supporting this theory show that children with Insulin Dependent Diabetes Mellitus (Type 1 or IDDM) have higher levels of these antibodies against cow milk proteins.[93] Still other studies have recognized that cow's milk may indeed trigger IDDM and have further shown a direct link between dairy consumption and Type 1 Diabetes.[94,95] As briefly mentioned above, dairy, like meat, is also implicated in cancer promotion. Specifically, dairy products are known to increase insulin-like growth factor-1 (IGF-1), a protein that stimulates cell growth and development but can also initiate cancer growth and accelerate aging.[96]

> ## Among the cancers associated with
> ## dairy consumption and IGF-1 production are
> ## breast, prostate, colon, small cell lung cancer,
> ## melanoma, and cancer of the pancreas.[97]

Many studies confirm this data, and we have chosen a few to share with you. The American Journal of Clinical Nutrition recently published a study that looked at whether childhood consumption of dairy was associated with incidence of cancer in adults. The study concluded that "A family diet rich in dairy products during childhood is associated with a greater risk of colorectal cancer in adulthood."[98] Another study published by the leading general medicine journal, The Lancet, observed that pre-menopausal women with high levels of IGF-1 had up to a seven-fold increase in breast cancer risk.[99] Finally, in a Harvard's Physicians Health Study, looking at over 20,000 men, researchers concluded that the consumption of dairy products and calcium are associated with a greater risk of prostate cancer.[100]

Another link between dairy and cancer is a consequence of cows being milked throughout their pregnancy, which results in their milk containing a very large load of estrogen. The average amount of estrone sulfate (which is converted to estrone and estradiol by the body) in milk from non-pregnant cows is 30pg/mL compared to 1,000pg/mL in pregnant cows (between 220-240 days of gestation).[101] And, milk and dairy products provide us with about 60-80% of the estrogen we consume.[102] It is well documented that certain cancers are estrogen-sensitive, so is it any wonder, then, that this increase in estrogen leads to these types of cancers (including breast, uterine, testicular, and prostate)?

> ## Last, but not least, dairy is laden with
> ## toxic and infectious agents.

Among dairy's leading toxins is dioxin, a byproduct of many industrial processes and one of the most carcinogenic compounds that exists in our environment. According to the EPA, of all of the animal products available to us, dairy provides us with the highest load of Dioxin.[103] This is due to bio-magnification (see Figure 9, Chapter 8). As for infectious agents, most of us are probably familiar with the more common outbreaks of E. coli, Salmonella, Botulism, and Foot and Mouth Disease. How many of you remember the Mad Cow Disease scare? But have you heard about Bovine Immunodeficiency Virus (BIV), Bovine Leukemia Virus (BLV), or Bovine Tuberculosis Virus? In the United States, about 40% of beef herds and 64% of dairy herds are infected with BIV.[104] And according to Hoard's Dairyman, the self proclaimed "National Dairy Farm Magazine," "most dairy herds (about 89% of them) are affected by BLV."[105] It should be noted that Bovine Leukemia Virus is closely related to HTLV-1, a virus that causes leukemia and lymphoma in humans. A study done by Dr. Gertrude Case Buehring and colleagues, at the University of California School of Public Health in Berkeley, looked at a population of people to see if they had BLV antibodies. Surprisingly, they found that 74% of their subjects tested positive.[106] Because most of these subjects did not have direct contact with the animals, it was deduced that they developed antibodies indirectly as a result of consuming beef and dairy products. In this study, the research could not determine with certainty whether the immune response was a result of infection or a reaction to dead viruses present in the eaten animals. However, another study by the same author found BLV DNA in human blood cells and BLV proteins in human breast tissue.[107] These results suggest that humans can indeed become infected with BLV. Note that we are not saying dairy causes leukemia or HIV, but we are saying that the above facts should be considered in evaluating whether or not to include dairy in your diet. As for Tuberculosis, according to the Center for Disease Control, it remains "one of the most widespread infectious diseases and is the leading cause of death due to a single infectious agent among adults in the world. *Mycobacterium tuberculosis* is the most common cause of human TB, but an unknown proportion of cases are due to *Mycobacterium bovis*."[108] Transmission occurs via direct contact with diseased cattle and farm workers or from consuming infected food products (particularly unpasteurized milk and dairy products). Although the greatest number of people affected are in developing countries, industrialized countries are not immune. As a matter of fact, the direct link between *Mycobacterium Bovis* in cows and tuberculosis in humans has been well documented in the scientific literature, even in industrialized countries.[109]

Doesn't pasteurization protect us?

Unlike sterilization, pasteurization does NOT kill all disease-causing microorganisms.

Rather, it reduces their numbers, making it less likely, but not impossible, for them to cause disease. In other words, pasteurization is not a cure-all, it does not protect us from all pathogens, and outbreaks associated with pasteurized products continue to occur.

The following are just a few examples of such outbreaks here in the United States:

1985 – Outbreak of *Salmonella typhimurium* in Illinois associated with pasteurized milk. 16,000 cases were confirmed but over 150,000 people became ill.[110]

1994 – Outbreak of Listeria monocytogenes in Illinois associated with chocolate milk consumption. Forty-five cases identified, four people were hospitalized.[111]

1994 – Outbreak of Salmonella enteriditis nation-wide associated with pasteurized ice cream. An estimated 224,000 people developed S. enteriditis gastroenteritis.[112]

1995 – Outbreak of Yersinia enterocolitica in Vermont and New Hampshire associated with bottled pasteurized milk. Ten cases were identified, three patients were hospitalized, and one underwent an appendectomy.[113]

2006 – Outbreak of *Campylobacter jejuni* in California associated with pasteurized milk. Fifty-two cases were confirmed although 1592 people became ill.[114]

2007 - Outbreak of *Listeria monocytogenes* infections in Massachusetts associated with pasteurized milk. Five cases were identified and three people died.[115]

After reading this, you may still struggle with the idea of eliminating dairy, but don't feel bad; you are not alone.

Dairy is an addiction, literally.

More specifically, in the process of digesting the dairy protein casein, substances called "casomorphins" are produced.[116] These casomorphins, particularly concentrated in cheese, activate the same receptors in our body as does morphine. In addition to giving us a euphoric sensation, some of these casomorphins have as much as 1/10 the pain-killing potency of morphine.[117] No wonder people have such a visceral response when they are asked to eliminate dairy, and specifically cheese. It would be akin to asking a heroin addict to stop using heroin. In all honesty (although this is by no means our recommendation), it is almost better to sprinkle morphine on your healthy plant food than to take it in the form of dairy – at least this way you will ensure that you get some nutrients with your drugs. The take-home message here is that, for most of us, we crave dairy (and especially cheese) not because it is delicious but because we are unknowingly addicted to it. And like any other addiction, withdrawing from this drug will not be easy. It will require time, patience, strength, and determination, but the successful elimination of this disease-promoting food will be worth its weight in gold (in this case, your health and well-being).

In summary, it seems that short of taste preference, dairy has no redeeming qualities, unless you are a young calf, of course. The question then becomes, is the taste worth its weight in heart disease, cancer, diabetes, infections, or obesity? That is up to you.

Take-home messages:

- Calcium is a mineral found in the earth and absorbed by plants.
- Animals acquire calcium by eating plants.
- The average calcium intake in most Western countries is 800-1000mg/day. This is 150%-200% MORE than the 500mg/day recommended by the World Health Organization.
- Problems with dairy (i.e., "liquid meat"):
  - High in protein
  - High in calories
  - High in fat
  - Contains cholesterol
  - Laden with toxins and infectious diseases
  - Major cause of food allergies
  - Increases risk of heart disease, diabetes, osteoporosis, and cancer, among others.
- Vitamin D is a hormone activated by sun exposure.
- Most of the vitamin D found in milk is added to it.
- Dairy does not help with weight loss; remember, its original function is to grow a 60 lb calf into a 600 lb cow.
- Pasteurization does not protect us from all pathogens.
- Casomorphins are produced in the process of breaking down dairy and ACT ON THE SAME RECPETORS, IN OUR BODY, AS MORPHINE.

Chapter 11: Fats and Oils

Did you know that the average American gets 30-40% of daily calories from fat and 15% from saturated fat?[118] This is double the already generous amount recommended by the American Heart Association (AHA). In fact, according to the AHA,

> "Saturated fat intake should not exceed
> 7% of total calories each day (with optimal levels
> less than 5%), and trans fat (agreed to be the most
> dangerous type of fat) intake should not exceed
> 1% of total calories each day."[119]

According to the National Academy of Sciences, there is no safe level of trans fat consumption. "There is a positive linear trend between *trans* fatty acid intake and total and LDL cholesterol concentration, and therefore increased risk of CHD (coronary heart disease), thus suggesting a Tolerable Upper Intake Level (UL) of zero." Although trans fats are primarily found in fried and processed foods, the National Academy of Sciences further recommends eliminating "foods, such as dairy products and meats, that (also) contain *trans* fatty acids."[120] Why isn't this message advertised as readily as the "golden arches" or those "got milk" white mustaches? Especially in light of the fact that,

> over the last 30 years, childhood obesity has tripled,
> and today two-thirds (66%) of adults are overweight,
> and of those, half (50%) are obese.[121,122]

Maybe, this message isn't advertised because it would threaten those companies whose livelihoods depend on Americans getting and staying fat; particularly, the fast food, meat, and dairy industries.

Are we telling you not to eat fats? No. On the contrary,

dietary fats, just like proteins and carbohydrates, are essential

for the body to perform a variety of important functions. The problem is not whether to incorporate fat into your diet; rather, the question is how much you add and what type of fat you are consuming. Dietary fats are divided into two categories: saturated fats that are solid at room temperature (mostly from animal products) and unsaturated fats that are liquid at room temperature (mostly from plants). The unsaturated fats are further divided into poly-unsaturated and mono-unsaturated fats. Dietary fats are made from a combination of these saturated and unsaturated fats (see Figure 10).

Figure 10 – A Breakdown of the Percentage of Saturated, Monounsaturated, and Polyunsaturated Fat in Various Oils

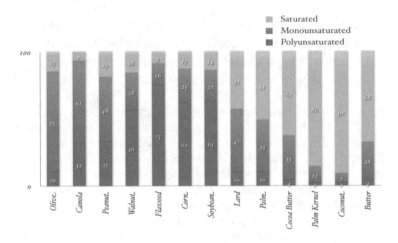

Of all the fats, there are only two essential fatty acids (EFAs) – that's right, only two! What does that mean? That means that these are the only two fats we must get from our foods; the rest our body can make on its own. What are these two essential fats, you might ask? They are omega-3 (or alpha-linolenic acid) and omega-6 (or linoleic acid), both polyunsaturated fats.

The only two essential fatty acids we need are omega-3 and omega-6.

This may not be news to many of you, especially in light of the recent EFA media hype. Some article titles you may have seen include: "Omega-3: Protect Your Heart with These Miracle Fats"; "Omega-3s: Fishing for Happiness"; "Intellect Doubles in Teens Who Eat Fish";

"Getting thin-on fats: The healthy, sure-fire way with omega oils", and so on. Although there are definite benefits to incorporating essential fatty acids into your diet, this is not a case where some are good and more are better. So, how much do we really need, where can we find them, and what are the pros and cons, if any?

According to the National Academy of Sciences,

> adequate daily intake of omega-3 fatty acids is
> 1.1 grams for women and 1.6 grams for men.[123]

This translates to between 1-3% of our daily calories or about ¼ to 1/3 of a teaspoon a day. Not very much at all and easy to attain with even the most basic plant-based diet. As a matter of fact, a 2000-calorie diet of lettuce alone gives you 7.7 grams of omega-3 fat.

True, most of us will not be eating 2000 calories of lettuce, but the take-home message is that we do not need to. As long as you are eating a plant-based diet rich in vegetables (especially leafy greens), fruits, nuts, seeds, legumes, and grains AND you are meeting your daily calorie requirement, you should be getting all of the EFAs you need. If, for whatever reason, you are still concerned, ground flax seeds (not the oil) and walnuts are two healthy sources for obtaining your EFAs. As a matter of fact, in ¼ cup of chopped walnuts there are 2.7 grams of omega-3 and 11.1 grams of omega-6, and in one tablespoon of ground flaxseed there is 1.6 grams of omega-3 and 0.4 grams of omega-6. Keep in mind that nuts are very calorie-dense (average of 2700 calories per pound), so use them sparingly, especially for those of you trying to lose weight.

Why do we recommend ground flaxseed and not whole flaxseeds or flax seed oil? Because ground flaxseeds are easily digested and provide the most nutritional benefit, including fiber, lignans, calcium, magnesium, iron, potassium, zinc, and folate. While whole flaxseeds also contain these nutrients, they are difficult to break up even with extensive chewing. Seeds that remain whole may not be properly digested. As for flaxseed oil, it is pure fat and lacks most of the nutrients and all of the fiber found in ground flaxseeds.

What about fish? Aren't fish and fish oils the perfect foods for obtaining Essential Fatty Acids (EFAs)? If you read our chapter about protein, then you know the answer to this question is NO! Fish is not a health food. Fish is high in cholesterol and loaded with contaminants from mercury to PCBs to dioxin (second only to dairy). Fish has also been linked to an increased risk of breast cancer.[124] (For more details please refer to Chapter 8 on Proteins.) But even more importantly, fish is not a **primary** source for obtaining EFAs. As a matter of fact,

fish get their essential fatty acids from the plants they eat

(remember that only plants can make EFAs). We could and should do the same and save ourselves the health risks.

Some might point out that we get DHA and EPA (two derivatives of omega-3, most readily used by the body, and particularly important for proper brain function and development) directly from fish. Is that also the case with plant sources for EFAs? True, fish already make the conversion from omega-3 to EPA and DHA for us so that when we eat fish, we get those derivatives directly. But again, at what price; especially in light of the fact that we can make the conversion ourselves. What about the assumption that our bodies are inefficient at converting omega-3 (i.e., alpha-linolenic acid or ALA) to EPA and DHA? Well, that depends on how we look at it and whom we talk to. If you talk to people selling supplements, they will tell you your body can't effectively convert ALA to EPA and DHA. Then they will push to sell you their line of drugs. But, press THEM a little further and they might tell you this really only applies to some people, in particular diabetics. The truth is that,

most of us eating a balanced, oil-free, whole foods diet with enough ALA could and should adequately convert ALA to EPA and DHA.[125]

The reason that many people on a typical American diet don't convert efficiently is not because their bodies are flawed. Rather, it is because they get too little ALA to begin with (and you can't adequately convert something you don't have enough of), they don't consume foods that are helpful in the conversion process (fruits and vegetables rich in magnesium, zinc, and vitamins C, B3, and B6) or because they eat other foods that inhibit an effective conversion process (including saturated fats, trans fats, hydrogenated fats, alcohol, and cholesterol). Another factor is consuming too much omega-6, which competes with omega-3 (ALA) for the enzymes required in the conversion process.

But, isn't omega-6 good for us? Going back to what we said earlier, some omega-6 is good for you, but more, in this case, is not better. Another important thing to consider is the ratio of omega-6 to omega-3. Omega-3 breaks down in our body into anti-inflammatory agents while omega-6 breaks down into both anti- and pro-inflammatory agents. When we maintain the proper ratios, these two important

EFAs work together to promote healthy brain functioning as well as protect us from diseases such as atherosclerosis (hardening of the arteries), heart attacks, strokes, cancer, and arthritis.

Ideally, we want our ratio of omega-6 and omega-3 to be between 1:1 and 4:1.

The American diet, whenever it does manage to squeeze in EFAs, overdoes the omega-6 (because of its prevalence in vegetable oils, processed foods, and meats) and neglects the omega-3. As a matter of fact,

in the United States today, the ratio of omega-6 to omega-3 is between 10:1 and 25:1.[126]

The problem with this is that omega-6 and omega-3, in order to be converted in our body, compete for the same enzymes.[127] An excessive amount of omega-6 means it will crowd out omega-3 at the receptor sites, creating an imbalance that then contributes to heart disease, cancer, inflammatory, and autoimmune diseases. Not convinced? Don't take our word for it; look at the data. In patients with heart disease, "a ratio of 4:1 was associated with a 70% decrease in total mortality. The lower omega-6 to omega-3 ratio (2.5:1) in women with breast cancer was associated with decreased risk (of recurrence). A ratio of 2-3:1 suppressed inflammation in patients with rheumatoid arthritis, and a ratio of 5:1 had a beneficial effect on patients with asthma, whereas a ratio of 10:1 had adverse consequences."[128]

Although our immediate response may be to increase our omega-3, really what we should be focusing on is decreasing our omega-6. Why? Because the problem here, for most of us, is not so much a deficiency of omega-3 (which is easily corrected by eating an oil-free, whole foods, plant-based diet or by adding one to two tablespoons of ground flaxseed to your daily diet), but an abundance of omega-6. Adding omega-3 without decreasing omega-6 will definitely improve your ratio but it will also increase your total fat intake. Remember that ratio (of omega-6 to omega-3) is only one ingredient in the recipe for health, the others being taking in the right fats (omega-3 and omega-6) and taking in the right quantities (omega-3 = 1.1 grams for a woman and 1.6 grams for a man, omega-6 = 5-10 grams for an average adult). Imagine you are baking an apple cake that calls for 2 cups of apples and one cup of sugar along with all of the other ingredients. Now, lets say you add 6 cups of apples, and to balance that you add 3 cups of sugar. Well, yes, you have gotten the right ratio of apples to sugar but what happened to your cake? All of the other ingredients stayed the same so really you end up with a heap of sugared apples and not much of a cake. The same process occurs in our bodies. We only need a small amount of EFAs; any excess upsets the body's natural balance. And what's more, that surplus gets saved and stored in our hips, thighs, bellies, and butts just like any other fat.

So, the goal becomes to decrease the omega-6 in your diet. This may prove slightly challenging on a typical American diet as, unlike omega-3, omega-6 is found abundantly in vegetable oils, processed foods, and meats (remember that these animals, like fish, get their omegas from the plant foods they eat).

One way to increase your omega-3, decrease your omega-6, AND get a healthy ratio of both is to incorporate more natural, whole, plant-based foods.

In this way you will bake the perfect "cake," as in the example above, with all of the right ingredients (vitamins, minerals, fiber, anti-oxidants, and essential fatty acids) in just the right amounts.

Where does olive oil fit in? It doesn't. For one thing, olive oil is composed mostly of mono-unsaturated fats, which are not essential. In fact,

to get enough omega-3 from olive oil, you would need to drink 8 ounces per day, that is one cup, 1900 calories, and 216 grams of saturated fat.[129]

Another interesting thing to note is that for all of its marketing, olive oil has as many poly-unsaturated fats as lard and far less of the essential omega-3 fats (the fats we should care about) than canola, peanut, walnut, flaxseed, corn, or soybean oil (see Table 10).

What about the polyphenols in olive oil; aren't those good for us? This again is another example of the reductionist theory where the olive oil Industry promotes polyphenols (because it is one of the few positive things about olive oil) just like the Dairy Industry promotes calcium (see Chapter 10). Polyphenols (plant sterols) are antioxidants believed to have various health benefits, from protecting the heart to preventing cancer. But, polyphenols are not exclusively found in olive oil, they are abundant in many fruits and vegetables (including apples, blueberries, cantaloupe, grapes, pears, broccoli, cabbage, kale, onions, etc.), so much so, that olive oil pales in comparison. For example, to get 30mg of polyphenols you need to have one tablespoon of olive oil (120 calories and 13grams of fat) or ten blueberries (8 calories and 0 grams fat).[130]

So, why all the hype? Because researchers noticed that people on a Mediterranean diet are generally healthier than people on an American diet. Since Mediterranean cuisine generally incorporates olive oil, people jumped to the conclusion that this oil must be a magical elixir. The message then became *add olive oil to your diet to become healthier*, a message that is certainly delicious to swallow. And that is indeed what many Americans did; they ADDED olive oil to their already fat-laden diet. Now, let's stop for a second and do the math. The recommended daily fat intake (a VERY generous recommendation) is less than 20-35% of our daily calories, with saturated fat being less than 7%. The average daily intake of fat in the United States is about 37%, with about 12% from saturated fat.[131] We are not mathematicians, but even we can see that adding ANY amount of fat (e.g., olive oil) to 37% and 12% will not get us under 20-35% or less than 7%.[132]

Okay, then where did we go wrong? Well, first of all, we bought into a very well delivered marketing hype. Even if pure oils provided us with a good source of omega-3, many other oils would be better choices for use than olive oil (see Figure 10). But more importantly, we didn't examine the data carefully enough. Yes, people on the Mediterranean diet are healthier and yes, they do use olive oil, BUT they also have a diet rich in fruits and vegetables and limited in meats, dairy, and fast foods (at least those that have not yet switched over to a Western Diet). There are two important take-home messages here. One, is that they base their diet on fruits, vegetables, and grains. These are the staples to which other foods are added in smaller amounts. Second, they use olive oil INSTEAD of saturated and trans fats (i.e., lard, butter, palm kernel oil) not in ADDITION to them. In this particular case, yes olive oil is the lesser evil. This is analogous to stapling your finger with a large staple gun (saturated and trans fats) versus a regular stapler (olive oil). Just because the smaller staple hurts less doesn't take away from the fact that it is hurting you. In the same way,

olive oil as a replacement for oils
high in saturated fat may be a better choice
but that does NOT make olive oil healthy.

In fact, olive oil still raises cholesterol and damages blood vessels, it just doesn't do it to the extent that the saturated fats do.[133,134]

Furthermore, a study that looked at olive oil's effect on blood flow showed that a single meal with olive oil caused increased vessel spasm and decreased blood flow.

Specifically, this study showed that when test subjects were fed the olive oil meal, their major blood vessels had a 31% decrease in blood flow![135] In effect, what is happening with this fatty meal is that the blood cells are clumping together, the circulation of blood is slowing down, and there is a reduction in the amount of oxygen available to tissues.[136] Our blood should be like water smoothly flowing through a pipe (our blood vessel). What happens after an oily fatty meal is that we have sludge-like oil running through those pipes. Now instead of a smooth steady flow we have a slow and sluggish flow. Considering that these "pipes" not only deliver nutrients to your entire body but also supply you with the oxygen you need to thrive and survive, what would you prefer to have running through them? If you are not sure, just try an oil-free, whole plant foods diet for a few weeks and see how much lighter you feel.

The bottom line is that the trends will change and there will always be the latest and greatest product on the market but,

> oil is oil, no matter what food it is extracted from
> (a soybean, an olive, a flax seed, or a coconut),
> and ALL oil is bad for you.

Case in point is coconut oil (the latest craze) and the purported benefits of its medium-chain fatty acids (MCFAs). Coconut oil is over 90% saturated fat and has the same detrimental effect on our cholesterol as eating butter.[137] Let us assume that the studies on MCFAs (still saturated fat) are accurate and, that these substances are indeed absorbed directly into the liver, are oxidized a little more quickly, have less of an effect on LDL (your bad cholesterol), and have the potential for weight loss. Now, let us subtract the amount of MCFAs (assuming that they have a beneficial effect) from the total amount of saturated fat. This still leaves us with 45% saturated fat, making coconut oil worse than lard, which only has 43% saturated fat. Does that now make lard a health food? Not by a long shot! The greatest irony in this coconut oil craze is that in many cases, the minimal amount of beneficial MCFAs in coconut oil are isolated and removed from the oil, to be used medicinally or in beauty products.[138] So in effect, you are getting all of the bad without any of the benefit, regardless of what oil you are using. Again, the take-home message is that,

oil, no matter where it comes from, is NEVER a health food.

In summary, you only need two types of fats from your diet, omega-3 and omega-6. All other fats (saturated, hydrogenated, trans, mono-unsaturated) at the very least are not helpful and at the very worst are extremely harmful (contributing to elevated cholesterol, clogging of the arteries, and heart disease). Eating a natural, whole foods, plant-based diet (or even just incorporating more fruits, vegetables, and grains into your diet) is your best bet to get not only the right amount but also the appropriate ratio of essential fatty acids. If that makes you nervous, and you need further insurance, then go ahead and incorporate a tablespoon or two of ground flaxseeds into your day.

For those of you on board and ready to limit or eliminate oils, here are some helpful cooking tips. First of all, go out and get yourself some non-stick pots and pans. These will greatly enhance your cooking experience. Next, throw out all of your cooking oils, butter, lard, margarine, etc. Replace these with non-fat liquids like vegetable broths, juices, vinegars (rice wine, balsamic, etc.) or sauces (tamari, barbeque, teriyaki, tomato, etc.). (For specific examples, see Appendix H.) You can use any of these to sauté, brown, or soften vegetables (see recipe section for instructions). Finally, when baking, substitute fruit, pumpkin, or tofu for oil, butter or margarine. If that isn't rich enough for you, you can also use a fat replacer (e.g., Wonderslim's fat and egg substitute). We have a few recipes in the back of this book that are delicious. Again, don't take our word for it; try them out for yourself. We have a feeling you won't regret it.

Take-home messages:

- "Saturated fat intake should not exceed 7% of total calories each day (with optimal levels less than 5%) and trans fat intake should not exceed 1% of total calories each day (even though ideally it should be 0%)."

- The average American gets 30-40% of daily calories from fat, 13% from saturated fat and 2% from trans fat.

- There are only two essential fatty acids (omega-3 or alpha-linolenic acid and omega-6 or linoleic acid), both polyunsaturated fats.

- Adequate daily intake of omega-3 is 1.1 grams for a female and 1.6 grams for a male.

- In ¼ cup of chopped walnuts there are 2.7 grams of omega-3 and 11.1 grams of omega-6, and in 1 tablespoon of ground flaxseed there is 1.6 grams of omega-3 and 0.4 grams of omega-6.

- Fish get their essential fatty acids by eating plants.

- We are able to convert omega-3 to EPA and DHA.

- Aim for an omega-6 to omega-3 ratio between 1:1 and 4:1 (not 10:1 to 25:1, as in the typical American diet).

- Olive oil is composed mostly of mono-unsaturated fats, which are NOT essential.

- To get enough omega-3 from olive oil, you would need to drink 8 ounces per day; that is 1 cup, 1900 calories, and 216 grams of fat!

- The traditional Mediterranean diet is healthy despite, and NOT because of, the olive oil.

- Coconut oil is over 90% saturated fat and has the same detrimental effect on your cholesterol as eating butter.

- Dietary fat (abundantly found in an oil-free, whole foods, plant-based diet) is essential for proper functioning, oil is NOT!

- Oil, no matter where it comes from, is NEVER a health food.

- Helpful tips for no-oil cooking:
    - Use non-stick pans
    - Sautee with non-fat liquids (vegetable broth, juice, vinegar)
    - Use oil-free sauces (tamari, BBQ, teriyaki, tomato)
    - In baking, substitute fruit, pumpkin, or tofu for oil, butter, or margarine.

Chapter 12: Carbohydrates

Okay, by now you might be tired of hearing what you can't eat...well, now some good news! This chapter is devoted solely to all the wonderful things you **can** eat. What? Under the heading of carbohydrates—are we out of our minds? Possibly, but NOT because we are telling you to eat carbs. Go ahead, read on.

So many of us have hopped on the carb-fearing bandwagon. We are worried that carbs are not nutritious, they are comfort foods, they contribute to diabetes, and they make us fat. In reality, carbohydrates can be our friends. In fact,

> carbohydrates are our body's most
> efficient source of energy,

the preferred energy for the brain, and the only energy for our red blood cells and certain kidney cells.[139] Furthermore, studies show that a low-fat, high-carbohydrate diet is associated with increased satiety, reduced calorie consumption, and decreased obesity.[140]

Having said that, not all carbohydrates are created equal. We have simple carbohydrates, complex carbohydrates, and "man-made" carbohydrates (processed and refined junk foods). Simple carbohydrates are made up of one or two sugars (glucose, fructose, sucrose, etc.) and are easily and swiftly absorbed by the body. The upside of this is that they provide the quickest source of energy to the body but the down side is that they cause our blood sugars to rise and then plummet equally as fast. Simple carbs can be further sub-divided into nutrient-filled, natural, simple sugars (e.g., some fruits and vegetables) and nutrient-depleted, processed and refined, simple sugars (e.g., candy, sodas, high fructose corn syrup, and table sugar). As their categories imply, the first group (nutrient-filled) contains important vitamins, minerals, and fiber while the second group (nutrient-depleted) is generally considered "empty calories" and devoid of most, if not all, nutrients. Complex carbohydrates are made up of a chain of three or more sugars and take longer for the body to break down and absorb. As a result, they provide a steadier source of energy as well as a more stable rise in blood sugar.

Complex carbs are found in vegetables, nuts, seeds, grains, and some fruits. Finally, the last category, "man-made" carbohydrates (processed and refined junk foods), are high in calories with minimal (if any) nutritional value. They can be either simple or complex and include cakes, cookies, jams, French fries, and potato chips.

Simple, complex, which are okay, which are not? This may indeed become confusing and therefore contribute to the carb-fearing craze. But, in reality it is very simple. The key is not to get bogged down with these classifications. Rather,

when eating carbohydrates, just choose natural, whole plant foods (including fruits, vegetables, whole grains, nuts, and seeds) as often as you can.

This will ensure that you get the balance of simple and complex carbohydrates that will provide you with the proper amounts of vitamins, minerals, and fiber, without getting the unnecessary calories and fat. In addition, you will also be choosing foods that are rich in proteins and contain all of your essential fats.[141] But, most importantly, you will be giving your body the fuel that it craves to run in the most efficient and effective manner.

Having trouble digesting this information? Let's try an analogy: imagine your body is a car trying to run on an empty gas tank; it wouldn't get very far, right? Okay, so you push it over to a gas station and you have a choice of gasoline: regular 87, plus 89, or premium 93. Now, *you* need to decide what kind of car you are. Are you a Yugo or a Rolls Royce? For most of us this is a no-brainer, as we would pick the Rolls over the Yugo every time. But to maintain that premium, sleek, and suave body, we need to fuel it appropriately. Although the Rolls Royce may run on regular gasoline, over time this would destroy the engine. The same concept applies to our bodies. We are meant to run on carbohydrates, our body's preferred energy source. When we do not have an adequate supply of carbohydrates, the body turns to other less efficient fuel sources like fats and proteins. These other sources of fuel should be saved for emergencies, but instead they have become the mainstay of the American diet. And, yes, we can break them down, but at what price? At the price of our body's thinking that we are in crisis (i.e., fasting or starving).

But, what about burning fat? Isn't that a good thing? Sure, if you have excess fat, getting rid of it is a key component in optimizing your health. The question now becomes how to lose the fat in a healthy and safe manner. You could fast or, as an even greater extreme, you could smoke crack, deplete your fat stores, and be thin as a rail, but that would not get you to achieve health, much less optimal health. You could also restrict your carbohydrates and/or your calories. This would cause your body to be unhappy on two counts: one, it would be starving (if you limit calories) and two, it wouldn't have its preferred energy source (if you limit carbohydrates). So, what does it do? It shifts into a default mode, a condition known as ketosis and definitely not our preferred state. Ketosis is the state where fat is broken down for energy. The byproducts of this type of fat breakdown are ketones. Excess accumulation of ketones stresses not only our kidneys, which ultimately need to excrete them, but also our livers that work to produce them and our bones that work to neutralize them (ketones are acidic). In fact, after just 3 weeks on a high-protein, low-carbohydrate diet people urinated 50% more calcium than they did prior to starting the diet.[142] Other side effects of ketosis include constipation, bad breath, fatigue, weakness, headaches, nausea, vomiting, and possibly even cognitive damage.[143] And worst of all, these side effects are endured to allow weight loss but in reality, the initial weight loss from a low-carb ketogenic diet is completely deceptive, as it is mostly water weight and not fat that is lost.

So, how should we get rid of fat?
The first step is NOT to add more fat.

Fat was an important form of energy for the survival of our ancestors. They needed this stored energy to prevent them from starving in times of famine. When was the last time we in the United States experienced famine? That being said, some fat is necessary in our diet. But, as we explained earlier (see Chapter11), only two of the fats are essential (omega-3 and omega-6), and you only need a few grams of these essential fats (1-3% of total calories). Also, you can get all the fat you need from eating a natural, whole foods, plant-based diet. For example, oats are 16% fat, garbanzo beans are 9% fat, and apples are 3% fat. The next step is to go ahead and add those carbohydrates. It is important to note that,

humans do NOT efficiently convert
carbohydrates to fat. In fact, humans burn off much
of the excess carbohydrates they consume as heat.[144,145]

For those of you working to lose weight, make vegetables the majority of your meal. To that, add starches (root vegetables, whole grains, and legumes) and/or fruits based on your preference. But make sure you are eating more than just vegetables, as eating only vegetables will ensure your failure. Why? Because, we cannot thrive on vegetables alone; they are too low in calories. If we tried, we would become calorie-starved, weak, tired, irritable, and unsatisfied. Our metabolism would slow down and our deprivation would go through the roof. The end result is probably all too familiar for many of us; we throw our hands up, say "the heck with this," and head straight to our nearest fast food restaurant or donut shop. This is a really important concept to grasp, so we will re-emphasize it:

YOU WILL NOT SUCCEED ON VEGETABLES ALONE. YOU MUST ALSO EAT STARCHES (root vegetables, whole grains, and legumes) AND/OR FRUITS.

The ratio of veggies to legumes to starches to fruits is up to you. Again, for those of you looking to rapidly lose weight, make your meal 2/3 vegetables and 1/3 fruits, legumes, and/or starches (based on your preference). For the rest of you on a more moderate weight loss plan, keep it half and half. You may also garnish (not gorge) your meals with nuts, seeds, and avocados, as these are natural, whole, and healthy sources of fat. The key is to find the combinations of these whole foods that satisfy you enough to stick with this diet and lifestyle for a lifetime.

The final step is to get up and move. We burn some energy when we are sedentary but not nearly enough to budge a scale. We have to engage in some form of physical activity. For one thing, our intrinsic calorie-counting mechanism, as well as the hormones responsible for appetite control, work more accurately when we are active.[146] Furthermore, not only is exercise good for our hearts and general well-being, it is an excellent way to burn our extra fat stores.

Still nervous? We are not surprised. What took so many years to ingrain in your heads will take some time to undo. So, don't be hard on yourself: take your time, just maintain an open mind and keep reading. What's important to understand is that, until recently, carbohydrates have been a significant part of our diet. In fact, we are genetically engineered to seek out sweet tastes via the taste buds that sit on the tip of our tongue. Some theorists believe this ability was selected for over the years as a survival benefit.[147] One idea being that sugary foods were quickly converted into energy and therefore made our ancestors better equipped to either face danger or run from it.

The problem today is several-fold. First, unlike our ancestors, most of us no longer eat to live, we live to eat. This in and of itself may not be terrible IF we ate the right foods. But, the reality is that we don't and, instead, our typical Western diet is laden with meat, dairy, fats, oils, and refined simple sugars (devoid of vitamins, minerals, fibers, proteins, and essential fats). Second, although a sweet tooth may have been advantageous to our ancestors, they satisfied it with fruit and **not** with chocolate bars, candies, ice cream or sodas. Not only are fruits healthier in that they have little fat and fewer calories, but they prevent over-consumption. If you don't believe that, see how many apples, oranges, grapefruits, or bananas you can eat. That is not the case for today's processed, refined, sugary foods. These

processed foods are far too easy to find, they are loaded with calories, fats, and other unhealthy ingredients (hydrogenated oils, high fructose corn syrup, artificial coloring and flavor, etc.), and they have a built-in mechanism to ensure that you over-consume.

This is in part because processed foods are more calorie-dense, as they are lacking much of the water and fiber (which contributes bulk but no calories) found in whole foods. In other words, by removing the fiber and water, the food becomes much more concentrated and therefore higher in calories and often lower in bulk (see Table 10 for more examples). In addition, remember that our hunger signals are not as accurate in response to foods higher in fat. So, together these factors cause the stretch of our stomach to no longer match up with our caloric intake, which impairs our satiation system and causes us to over-consume (see calorie currency discussion in Chapter 1).

Table 10 - Calorie Density Table

WHOLE FOODS	CALORIES per POUND		MORE PROCESSED FOODS	CALORIES per POUND
Cabbage	100	→	Fast Food Coleslaw	700
Tomatoes	150	→	Sun Dried Tomatoes	1150
Apricots	200	→	Dried Apricots	1100
Grapes	300	→	Raisins	1350
Bananas	400	→	Banana Chips	2350
Sweet Potato	400	→	Sweet Potato Fries	1100
Brown Rice	500	→	Brown Rice Flour	1500
Corn	500	→	Corn Chips with Oil	2500
Olives	600	→	Olive Oil	4000
Avocado	750	→	Avocado Oil	4000

What's worse is that most processed carbs are "man-made" carbs, which make up a large part of the American diet. Not only are these "man-made" carbs "empty calories" lacking mostly, if not entirely, of any nutritional value, but they actually do harm in our bodies. Among their detrimental effects, they rapidly raise our blood sugars, causing our pancreas to secrete more insulin. Elevated insulin levels do two things: one, help mobilize fat into fat cells and two, remove sugars from the blood, causing our blood sugar to plummet. Add to this the fact that many of the common carbs in the American diet are also loaded with fat (potato chips, cookies, ice cream, etc.), which our bodies store very efficiently. These factors cause us to gain weight and leave us feeling hungry, tired, and craving more sugary junk foods. And this is how the vicious cycle is established: we eat these refined sugars, we get a "high," we crash, we seek our next "fix." This high that we are feeling is not just a subjective feeling, it is an actual chemical change that occurs in our brains.[148] We have engaged the dopamine-pleasure cycle that was discussed in Chapter 1. To recap, our brain understands that we are obtaining pleasure from eating these foods and, in response, releases dopamine that then reinforces this sense of pleasure. Our bodies and brains are smart and very adaptive so they quickly learn that eating these foods will reproduce these pleasurable sensations. And this is how the addiction begins.

So, what is the answer?

The answer is to make carbohydrates our friends.

How friendly you get depends on what your goals are for health, weight loss, and well-being. Our recommendation is to use the Food Continuum[34] as your guide. Ideally, you want to aim for an "A" range diet. Again, you can achieve this goal in several ways. The easiest and most helpful is to follow the 3-Phase Eating Plan (see Appendix B for more information) with every meal. In this manner, you ensure that you get your A+ foods in (with course 1 and course 2) prior to moving down the continuum with course 3. Another option is to choose to average an A over the course of your day. In this manner, you have more flexibility with each meal in that you could have a B lunch and then an A or A+ breakfast and dinner. For example, having oatmeal with fruit for breakfast (an A+), a veggie burger for lunch (a B), and tomato vegetable whole-grain pasta (no oil) for dinner (an A). You could also break up your meals to have a small B or C component combined with a larger A or A+ component. As an example, you could have a veggie burger on a whole grain bun with a large side of greens (make sure the greens constitute at least half of your meal portion), or you could have Thai peanut noodles with a large side of steamed broccoli (make sure the broccoli constitutes at least half of your meal portion). The point is that the options and the combinations are limited only by your creativity and motivation. For some recipe ideas, see Appendix I.

Take-home messages:

- Carbohydrates are our body's most efficient, and preferred, source of energy.

- A low-fat, high-carbohydrate diet is associated with increased satiety, reduced calorie consumption, and decreased obesity.

- Do NOT get bogged down with carbohydrate classifications (simple versus complex). Rather, when eating carbohydrates choose natural whole plant foods (fruits, vegetables, whole grains, nuts, and seeds) to get the proper balance that you need.

- Do NOT eat vegetables alone. YOU MUST INCLUDE STARCHES (root vegetables, whole grains, and legumes) AND/OR FRUITS IN YOUR MEALS!

- Remember to include daily physical activity (which helps stimulate your metabolism and regulate your appetite).

- Refined, processed foods have a built-in mechanism to ensure you over-consume.

- Eating refined sugars causes you to enter the dopamine-pleasure cycle where you get a "high," you crash, and then you seek your next "fix."

- When eating, aim for an "A" range diet by:
    o Following the 3-Phase Eating Plan
    o Averaging an "A" over the course of the day

Chapter 13: Supplements

"Can I get that to go?" "Do they have a drive thru?" "I only have a minute or two." Any of these sound familiar? For many of us, this day-to-day rush against the clock has become our baseline. We live for immediate gratification because we just don't have the time to wait around for events to naturally unfold. We eat in our cars or "on the go" instead of sitting for a meal, we shop on-line instead of heading to a store, and we take supplements instead of consuming the healthy whole foods where the nutrients originate.

For some of us, this is the best we can do; but for most of us, we can and should strive to do better. The general idea is that whenever possible we should eat the nutrients we need from the source, not supplement with a pill. Just think about it; why put something artificially manufactured into your body when the natural form, found in whole foods, is available to you and is better and safer for you?

> Nature has provided us with an abundance
> of natural whole foods. These foods come perfectly
> packaged with proteins, carbohydrates, fats,
> vitamins, minerals, and fibers.

Not only are these nutrients readily and abundantly available in these whole foods, but they are delivered in the right balance and proportion. Compare this to supplements, which are manipulated and isolated and function individually rather than collectively in our bodies. Think of your car, and then imagine trying to drive it with just a steering wheel, a tire, and a windshield; you wouldn't get very far, right? When we eat a diet rich in whole foods, we get a balanced variety of all the nutrients that we need in their proper proportions. They are then appropriately metabolized in our bodies and allow us to function optimally, giving us the whole car. Supplements, on the other hand, rather than delivering the entire car (with all of its gadgets and gizmos in the right proportions), deliver a steering wheel and an engine here, two tires and a body there, and so on. Unlike this analogy, in which obtaining parts of a car instead of the car itself may be annoying and inconvenient, the fragments delivered by

supplementation may actually cause us harm.

How does this happen? Like we said before, supplements introduce not only a synthetic product into the body but do so in artificial amounts. Often these doses are much higher than our actual needs. So, what happens is we get an additional amount of one, or even several, compounds that then upsets our body's natural balance? Unfortunately, this imbalance does not just result in expensive urine. For example, iron supplementation is often used to treat certain anemias. But, taking too many iron supplements may lead to overconsumption and iron poisoning, which can damage the stomach, the digestive tract, and the liver.[149] This is of particular concern because iron is found in many vitamin supplements and may be over-consumed when pills are combined. Another example is DHA, a long-chain form of omega-3 fatty acid. Some forms of DHA supplementation have been shown to increase DPAn-6. And DPAn-6 has been shown to retroconvert to arachidonic acid, a pro-inflammatory substance potentially harmful in excess. Furthermore, excess DHA gets saturated, and we all know the dangers of saturated fat.[150] And iron and DHA are not alone; overconsumption of calcium was associated with increased risk of heart attack, stroke, and death as well as kidney stones and kidney damage.[151] Excess magnesium can lead to muscle weakness and heart damage.[152] Too much vitamin A can result in seizures, liver damage, and even bone loss and osteoporosis.[153] Vitamin A, beta-carotene, and vitamin E all have been shown to increase mortality, and so on.[154]

The take-home message is that these supplements are not benign, and as a result, we should treat them like medications rather than an expensive insurance policy.

As medications, they should be used as a last resort for people who are unable to consume, absorb, or properly metabolize the natural forms of these nutrients and have proven deficiency diseases. And even when these *medications* are to be used, you should make sure you are appropriately informed and completely understand not only all the risks but also, the accuracy of the benefits reported. For example, for many people it is a no brainer to take folic acid supplements when trying to have a baby, but why do they "need" this supplement? Folic acid supplementation has been shown to significantly reduce neural tube defects (NTD), a deformity involving spinal cord development, in babies by 50%.[155] This statistic alone is enough for women to take the supplement without question and may also validate their judgment of anyone who chooses not to take the supplement as a negligent mother.

But, what happens when we delve a little deeper? Let us begin by finding out how likely it is to have a baby with a NTD in the first place. Studies show that if a woman does not take folic acid supplementation, her risk of having a baby with a NTD is 2 in 1000 (some sources even say this number is as few as 4-10 in 10,000).[156] In other words, if 1000 women choose NOT to supplement with folic acid, 998 of them will still have a normal baby and 2 of them will have a baby with a NTD. So, the reality is that the risk of having a baby with a NTD is small to begin with. Now, what happens when we supplement with folic acid? If a woman does supplement with folic acid then her risk of having a baby with a NTD decreases to 1 in 1000.[157] Which means that if 1000 women take folic acid, now 999 of them will have a normal baby and only 1 will have a baby with a NTD. In other words, taking folate results in only 1 extra woman out of 1000 (who all would have to take the pill with its potential risks) avoiding having a baby with a NTD while the other 999 women taking the supplement will see no benefit.

Does a 1 in 1000 risk reduction sound impressive to you? Maybe not, but 50% risk reduction probably does. The fact is, in this case, they are saying the same thing. Out of those 1000 women, instead of 2 women having a baby with a NTD the risk is reduced to 1 woman having a baby with a NTD, and 1 is 50% of 2. So that is how the data is manipulated to give us numbers that will impress us (50% reduction) versus numbers that won't (a decrease from 2/1000 to 1/1000).

That being said, are we telling you not to take folic acid? No! Even if the potential for a NTD is incredibly low, who among us wants to be that 1 mother who pays the price, especially, when taking folic acid is such an easy thing to do. Our concern is that taking folate supplements is not necessarily benign. In fact, one study suggested that women taking high doses of folate supplements throughout pregnancy may be more likely to die from breast cancer in later life than women not taking folate supplements.[158] So, rather than take a pill, let's think about it: where does folic acid come from? Well, folate or "foliage" is found naturally in plants and is supplied in abundance on a whole-plant-food diet. It is not found in animal products, processed foods, and oils, which constitute the majority of the typical American diet.

Why not then feed your baby, not only the folate it needs, but also the other vitamins, minerals, phytochemicals, and fiber that come in whole plant foods? Especially when, like we have said before, supplements are not benign. Folic acid is no exception. Noted side effects include abdominal cramps, diarrhea, nausea, gas, bloating, difficulty sleeping, irritability, and seizures.[159] Although none of these are fatal, they are certainly inconvenient and uncomfortable to experience, especially when it is completely unnecessary. By eating a whole foods, plant-based diet, mothers can provide their babies with a sufficient amount of folic acid without having to subject themselves to the nasty and potentially harmful side effects of supplementation.

Moving on, another common concern to validate the use of supplements is that our soil has been depleted and therefore our foods are no longer giving us the nutrients we need. But, do we really need to worry about soil depletion? This may be a valid concern for people who are getting their fruits and vegetables solely from their own backyard. However, this is not the case in the United States where we can get fruits and vegetables from around the world. Even if you only buy locally grown food, you can purchase produce from a variety of farms within a given region. In this manner, it is possible to compensate for any deficiencies. Another important consideration is that even if we only ate from one area and it was deficient in certain minerals, that does not mean there is a complete absence of that mineral, rather it means that there is just less of it than average. If the soil were completely devoid of a mineral, then the plants wouldn't grow either. So for example, if a particular area of soil only had 75% of the amount of iron compared to the average soil iron levels, that would still be okay. That's because we generally do not just eat enough to achieve 100% of the Dietary Reference Intake (DRI). Rather, if we eat a whole foods, plant-based diet, we usually eat well over that amount. So, if we normally eat double the DRI (often we consume even more than that just by meeting our caloric needs) then instead of achieving 200% we would achieve 150% - which is still 50% more than we actually need! This is especially so if we eat primarily whole foods to meet our caloric needs, as nature intended. Finally, at baseline, our intestines only absorb a fraction of the vitamin/mineral content of a particular food. Interestingly, the gut becomes more or less efficient at this absorption process based on an individual's need.[160] In this manner, nature has put in place many fail-safes to ensure that we get what we need. For example, if we need 500mg of calcium and we are getting 1500mg, our body will try to block some of that absorption. On the other hand, if we are only getting 500mg then our body will maximize our absorption to make sure we take in all of the calcium. Either way, the body's goal is to get 500mg.

If we really want to help ourselves along,

> ## rather than concern ourselves with supplements,
> ## we should focus on optimizing all aspects of our health
> ## since one area often affects another.

For example, rather than debate over supplementing calcium we should focus on getting enough sunlight to optimize our vitamin D levels. This is because research has shown that people with optimum vitamin D levels were able to absorb over TWICE as much calcium from the same meal as those with deficient vitamin D levels.[161]

What about a multivitamin? Doesn't that deliver a balanced composition of nutrients? First of all, a multivitamin cannot substitute for the abundance and assortment of antioxidants and phytochemicals available in natural whole foods. Second, in an effort to confer additional (and to date unproven) benefits, many multivitamins contain isolated nutrients at much higher doses than their daily-recommended amount. This can upset our body's natural balance and end up hurting rather than helping us. Finally, as concluded by the U.S. Preventive Services Task Force, there is insufficient evidence to support the use of vitamins (including a multivitamin) in the prevention of illnesses such as heart disease and cancer.[162] If we give supplements some thought, it makes absolute sense that,

> ## vitamin and mineral supplements
> ## cannot cure illnesses such as heart disease and cancer.
> ## Why? Because, for the most part, these are diseases
> ## of excess and not of deficiency.

They result from too much fried, junk, or fast foods, a sedentary lifestyle, and general apathy about preventive healthcare. We cannot expect to shovel junk into our bodies without consequence. We have to realize that in doing so, we are building up plaque in our arteries, raising our blood sugars and blood pressures, increasing our weight and promoting cancer cell growth. And then, we actually expect that one little daily multivitamin will somehow be a magic bullet to erase or neutralize the damage we do to our bodies every time we eat. This would be like cutting our hand three or more times a day and then applying a band-aid at the end of the day. Really, the band-aid is doing very little, if anything, for us. In fact, the band-aid might even impede our healing, and thus cause us harm. The truth is that until we stop cutting our hand, we will not be healed. The same applies to our diets and multivitamins. We cannot use supplements as a cure-all, instead we have to change our diets, our lifestyles, and our habits to incorporate better health and well-being. This is the only way to prevent illnesses like heart disease, diabetes, and cancer.

So, should we avoid all supplements? No, that is not what we are saying. Rather, we are telling you not to take supplements casually and/or as a replacement for a healthy diet and lifestyle. Like we stated before, treat supplements like medications and take them as a last resort only if you are truly deficient and unable to obtain, absorb, or metabolize the original source. Having said that, there are two exceptions. The first, is vitamin B12. This is the one vitamin that cannot be obtained sufficiently from today's plant-based diet. Why? Not because we need to eat animal products to obtain it. In fact, even adding animal products isn't always enough to replace B12.[163] The reason for this is that,

neither plants nor animals naturally synthesize B12.

Vitamin B12 is made from bacteria. Animals consume dirt (full of bacteria) with their plants and water, accumulate B12, and then become a source of the vitamin for humans. Let us re-emphasize, because it is very important: animals get their B12 by eating unwashed plants and non-chlorinated water (the dirt and water contain the bacteria that make B12). We, on the other hand, rarely eat anything unwashed and, therefore, in our quest to be clean, we remove the dirt (containing B12-producing bacteria) from our foods. This sanitary approach certainly has its benefits, as it has decreased our exposure to parasites and other pathogens. As a result, it is our educated guess that taking B12 supplementation is better than drinking/eating dirty foods. Vegans and vegetarians, especially, should supplement vitamin B12 (the Dietary Reference Intake is 2-3ug per day, although some people may need to take more).

Vitamin D is the second supplement we recommend to some of our patients. The importance of obtaining sufficient amounts of vitamin D should not be ignored as vitamin D is essential for optimum health. In fact, low levels of vitamin D are associated with increased rates of cancer, heart disease, and even mortality.[164] Unlike vitamin B12, however,

vitamin D can and should be obtained
through natural sources, namely the sun.

In fact, studies on vitamin D supplementation have shown an increase in blood levels of vitamin D but no significant benefit otherwise. For example, a meta analysis showing an almost negligible improvement in mortality with vitamin D supplementation concluded that "Population-based, placebo-controlled randomized trials with total mortality as the end point should be organized to confirm these findings."[165] In other words, better research needs to be done before making any recommendations about supplements improving important outcomes, such as mortality. This is especially so in light of the fact that vitamin D supplementation is not risk-free and has been associated with an increased risk of problems, such as kidney stones.[166] This is not a risk when we get our vitamin D from the sun.

But isn't sun exposure harmful and doesn't it cause cancer?

> Sun exposure, unlike sun **over**-exposure
> (which does cause skin damage and has been linked
> to cancer), has actually been shown to be
> beneficial to our health.

In fact, in a study done on indoor, outdoor, and mixed (both indoor and outdoor) workers, it was the mixed workers who had the least amount of skin cancer.[167] So it appears that some sun exposure is protective against cancer. Furthermore sunlight, unlike vitamin D supplements, is known to elevate mood, improve cognitive function, and help in the treatment of depression.[168]

We realize, however, that certain work environments as well as geographical limitations (with a low UV index) may make it difficult to get adequate sun exposure. For those people whose life circumstances prevent them from obtaining adequate sunlight, you should check your vitamin D levels, and if low, consider two options. One, UVB tanning booths and two, supplements. Remember these options are both distant seconds to sunlight exposure. Although tanning booths are more similar to sunlight as far as how we normally produce vitamin D, some people prefer to use supplements and that is their prerogative. If using a tanning booth be sure that it emits not just UVA light, as that will not raise vitamin D levels despite its ability to tan the skin. Also, since the UV index in a tanning booth is high (around 8-10 in an average tanning booth), be careful to avoid overexposure and the resulting skin damage. We make these recommendations because at this point it is our best guess that for those people who have a vitamin D insufficiency (levels between 20-30ng/mL) or deficiency (levels less than 20ng/mL) and are unable to obtain adequate sunlight exposure, the benefits of tanning and supplementation may outweigh the risks of low vitamin D levels.

For everyone else, make sure to:

1) Get out in the sun at least three to four days a week for about 10 to 15 minutes (this may vary depending on skin type and UV index, for more information go to http://www.exsalus.com/Site/H_I_4_Vitamin_D.html);
2) Expose as much skin as you can (ideally face, arms, legs, and even torso if possible); and
3) Make sure you go out when the UV index is 3 or greater (to check your local UV index on any given day go to www.epa.gov).

Beyond these two exceptions of vitamin B12 and sometimes vitamin D, we do not see a need for vitamin or mineral supplementation in a generally healthy individual. For those of you still hesitant to throw away the supplements, we encourage you to take advantage of our online nutritional analysis. Through this analysis of your average diet, we can determine what nutrients you are getting in sufficient amounts and what nutrients you are deficient in, based on the DRI (Dietary Reference Intake). Furthermore, if any deficiencies are noted, we can make recommendations on how to supplement your diet with whole foods (high in those particular nutrients) rather than with pills.

Take-home messages:

- **Whenever possible, we should get our nutrients from the whole food source rather than supplement with a pill.**

- **Nature has provided us with foods that are perfectly packaged with proteins, carbohydrates, fats, vitamins, minerals, and fibers.**

- **Supplements introduce not only a synthetic product into the body but do so in artificial amounts (often higher than our actual need).**

- **Supplements are not benign and should be treated like medication (taken as a last resort by people who are truly deficient and/or unable to obtain, absorb, or metabolize the original source).**

- **A multivitamin CANNOT substitute for the abundance and assortment of antioxidants and phytochemicals available in natural whole foods.**

- **The two exceptions:**
  - ○ **Vitamin B12 – especially for vegans and vegetarians**
    - ▪ **Vitamin B12 is made by bacteria.**
    - ▪ **Animals get their B12 from these bacteria.**
  - ○ **Vitamin D ONLY for those people unable to obtain it naturally through sun exposure.**

Chapter 14: Before You Begin

We have spent many chapters emphasizing the importance of a healthy diet in obtaining and maintaining optimal health. We have given you many dos and don'ts and have hopefully satisfied your curiosity as to why. Now, we would like to spend some time focusing on the "how." Specifically, we want to show you how to implement the Exsalus Health Program.

STEP 1: Identify your goals.

The idea is to determine what you need to do to make this diet taste delicious and make your new lifestyle feel fantastic. Examine where you are on the Optimum Health Continuum, decide where you would like to be, and then choose a realistic goal for your initial transition. Again, this is an individual assessment and requires you to be honest. You must take into account all of your rate-limiting steps, such as time, finances, support structure, etc. Then, figure out the steps necessary to successfully manage these challenges. Notice, we didn't say overcome – that is because it may not be realistic to overcome some of these hurdles (at least not right now), but that doesn't mean you should not get started. For example, your job may be extremely time consuming, and unless you have the luxury to quit or find a replacement job (which most of us don't) then your job will not go away (no matter how much and how hard you wish it to). So, your goal becomes to manage and work with, and around, your job schedule. Some suggestions include:

1)   Take one or two evenings a week or one weekend day and cook several dishes to refrigerate or freeze. These meals could then become healthy lunches for work.
2)   Park (or get dropped off) several blocks from work or take the stairs instead of the elevator whenever possible.
3)   Pack tennis shoes and use half of your lunch break to go for a walk.

4)   See if a friend or two want to commit to trying this program with you and/or take turns bringing in healthy lunches to work.

These are only a few recommendations for "managing" your job and its constraints on your time. We encourage you to complete the worksheet in Appendix D to identify your hurdles and come up with strategies to better prepare for and handle these challenges. The following chart includes an example to help you get started.

Table 11 – Identifying Your Challenges Worksheet

Rate-limiting step	Strategy 1	Strategy 2	Strategy 3
Ex. No time for cooking	Find one or two evenings or a weekend day and make several dishes that you can refrigerate and freeze for the week	Create a buddy system with a friend/co-workers and share the cooking. For example, take turns with four other co-workers where each member is responsible for bringing five servings of a healthy lunch. This way you only have to make one lunch a week.	Find restaurants willing to accommodate your dietary needs and buy meals from them.

For those of you questioning the usefulness of completing this chart, the idea here is to keep you one step ahead of yourself as well as accountable to yourself. We all have rough days and we all face obstacles. Unfortunately, some of us buckle under the stress and turn to our comforting, yet extremely unhealthy, habits (i.e. junk food, smoking, alcohol, etc.). We have found the best way to avoid traveling down that unhealthy road is to be prepared.

> By identifying your challenges and
> planning your management of them,
> you have an opportunity to jump over
> rather than crash into your hurdles.

STEP 2: Develop a meal plan

The goal here is not just to plan out your meals for the week but also to enable you to plan ahead (see Appendix E). If you plan all the meals you will have for the week, you can make one big shopping list and buy all of the ingredients in one shopping trip. Furthermore, if you have the opportunity, you can prepare several of the meals at a convenient time and store them in your fridge or freezer so they can be readily available to you. The most important function of the meal plan, however, is to make sure that you include enough rich foods, snacks, and desserts to make this a meal plan you look forward to.

Remember that what you eat on Monday, Tuesday, and Wednesday affects what you eat on Friday, Saturday, and Sunday.

In other words, the craving you have on Friday and the resulting binge on Saturday may simply have been due to having only carrot sticks and broccoli on Monday, Tuesday, and Wednesday. Do not, we repeat, DO NOT fill out the meal plan with just salads and steamed vegetables. That is not a sustainable diet and though you may lose weight in the short term, you will ultimately become extremely deprived and unhappy. This deprivation will lead to failure, and in our experience, people either stray from the diet temporarily or leave it completely. Remember, the idea is that

when eating a low-fat, whole foods, plant-based diet, you do not need to restrict calories.

That is because, these low-fat, whole plant foods are what your body thrives on and they are the foods that provide the correct "calorie currency" that will appropriately shut off your hunger signals (see Chapter 1). As such, you do not need to interfere by, for example, eating less and exercising more. This would be as detrimental as breathing less and exercising more. Trust yourself and trust your body, even if at this point it is difficult to do.

So, go ahead and make your meal plan palatable and satisfying by including plenty of starches (whole grains and root vegetables), some richer "seasonings" (nuts, seeds, or avocados), oil-free sauces, snacks, and desserts. Remember to balance your meals and create your 3-Phase Eating Plan (see Appendix B). Although the third course meal is optional, you want to make sure that you include enough of these foods over the course of the week to prevent you from feeling deprived. At the same time, however, you do not want to overindulge in these foods and may even choose to save them for times when you feel like "emotionally eating" or are feeling deprived. For those of you on the weight loss program, this notion of "saving" your richer foods may especially apply to you, and will help you more rapidly achieve your weight loss goal.

We have included a sample meal plan on the next page (see Figure 11) and encourage you to go to Appendix E to fill out your own chart. A good rule of thumb is to fill out your meal plan with the 3-Phase Eating Plan in mind. As such, make sure you include course 1 (your "multivitamin" or vegetables) and course 2 (your "filler" of whole, unprocessed foods such as grains, legumes, and root vegetables). The reasons for this are to: 1) get your nutrients in (remember nutrients first), and 2) fill up on these low-calorie, low-fat foods before indulging in your optional third course.

For those of you who travel or eat out a lot, don't panic.

You can still create an effective meal plan working around your schedule. If you are traveling, one option is to plan, make, and freeze your meals so that you can take them with you. This may seem weird at first, but it makes traveling so much less stressful as you know you will always have your food available to you. If this is not viable and you are relegated to eating out, here are some tips to help you navigate the restaurant world:

1)   Whenever possible, actively participate in the restaurant choice. For example, Asian cuisine - where you can get steamed rice and vegetables (steamed or stir-fried in no oil or sauces with very little oil), Mexican cuisine, where you can get a corn tortilla with guacamole and salsa on top of rice and beans (ask for whole beans without lard), and health food restaurants, which are generally more accommodating with menu modifications (check the Internet for vegan cuisine in your area).

2)   If you know ahead of time that you are going out to a place with little to no healthy choices, eat before you go. This way you will be satiated, able to order something light, and not be tempted to fill up on the unhealthy foods around you.

3)   Get clarification on ingredients (especially hidden ones like buttering of rice and breads, chicken broth and oil in soups, lard in beans, oil in sauces and salsas, and eggs in Asian foods).

4)   Do not be afraid to ask for a change in the menu or let the waiter know your dietary restrictions. Be sure to ask for their recommendation—you will be surprised at what a restaurant is willing to do to help you if you only ask (e.g., creating sauces with little

or no oil, steaming instead of frying). Sometimes it helps to explain to them how to prepare your dish without oil (for example sautéing with only the oil-free sauce, be that a bean sauce, a garlic sauce, soy sauce, etc.).

Figure 11 - Sample Meal Plan

	Monday	Tuesday	Wednesday	Thursday	Friday	Saturday	Sunday
Breakfast							
	Oatmeal with apples and berries, (2 tbsp) ground flax seeds	Smoothie (greens and fruit of your choice), 1-2 tbsp flax seeds optional	Watermelon (1/2-1 medium watermelon)	Large bowl of fruit and 2 whole grain blueberry pancakes	Smoothie (greens and fruit of your choice), 1-2 tbsp flax seeds	A large bowl of berries with ½ cup of oatmeal	Tofu scramble with LOTS of veggies and oil-free hash browns
Lunch							
	Bowl of raw broccoli with peanut sauce, potatoes dipped in cashew sauce, apple with +/-almond butter	Bowl of salad (lettuce, tomatoes, artichokes, onions, carrots, lime-juice, agave, nutritional yeast), black bean soup topped with crushed oil-free baked corn chips	Bowl of sautéed broccoli with peanut sauce, brown rice and beans on corn tortilla with salsa and guacamole, date/nut balls	Large salad (cabbage, cucumbers, tomatoes, , radishes, onions, peppers, mushrooms, balsamic vinegar dressing), oil-free hummus, baked falafel balls, pita bread, apple +/- almond butter	Bowl of carrot sticks, hearty dal soup (lentils, garbanzo beans, tomatoes, potatoes, onions, chard), bowl of puffed rice cereal with oat milk	Brown rice vegetable sushi, vegetable soup topped with oil-free baked corn chips, mango	Sweet potato dipped in oil-free hummus, cooked greens (kale, chard, spinach) dipped in peanut sauce, 2 date/nut balls
Dinner							
	Fresh asparagus sautéed in vegetable broth, crusted baked potatoes with salsa, slice of homemade vegetable pizza, piece of homemade carrot cake	Brussels sprouts and shallots sautéed in soy sauce and veggie broth, portabella mushrooms (sautéed in soy ginger sauce) on a sprouted whole grain bun, frozen banana with +/- peanut butter	Bowl of broccoli dipped in peanut sauce, bowl of vegetables sautéed in Korean BBQ sauce over brown rice, chilled mango slices	Cauliflower soup with peas, salad (cucumbers, tomatoes, onions), brown rice pasta with oil-free pesto, banana ice cream with or without some peanut butter mixed in	Bowl of sautéed greens in peanut sauce, lentil dish (lentils, peas, onions, garlic, tomatoes, spices) over brown rice, oil-free chocolate sorbet butter	Bowl of vegetable soup, lentil burgers and baked sweet potato fries, date/nut balls	Kale salad with peanut dressing, quinoa salad (quinoa, scallions, celery, peas, carrots, walnuts, dried cranberries), piece of home-made lasagna, frozen grapes

5)   If you can't find an entrée, order several appetizers or side dishes (like a dry baked potato or dry hash browns, vegetables, rice without butter, salad with no dressing or dressing on the side, etc.). Then you can use barbeque sauce, mustard, ketchup, salsa, or other condiments to flavor the dish to your liking.

6)   MOST IMPORTANTLY, know that sometimes all you can do is your best. In these situations, your meal may not be "perfect" but that too is okay, as long as it is the exception in your diet and not the rule.

STEP 3: Keep a food diary

The purpose of the Food Diary is to keep you mindful of what you are consuming while giving you a source to refer to if you are not progressing as quickly or as significantly as you would like (see Appendix F).

To be successful with the Food Diary,
you must be as honest and as thorough as you possibly can,
which means including every morsel, taste, nibble,
or bite that enters your mouth.

You can also include how you were feeling before, during, and after a meal, how satisfying the meal was, and whether you were satisfying a craving or temptation. Assess the diary once a week and use its information to create your new meal plan. This part is trial and error and over time you will find your groove. For example, if you felt deprived, include some richer meals. If certain foods didn't settle well, exclude them for the week and observe what happens. If you found yourself craving certain foods, try to make a healthy version of those foods. This last point is particularly important because

we all experience cravings.

Rather than ignore these craving using willpower, try to approach them with a sense of excitement. By this we mean challenge yourself to create these foods in a healthy manner. Instead of oil or other unhealthy fats, substitute avocados, olives, seeds, or nuts (whole, crushed, pureed, etc.) to add richness. And rather than using processed white flour, use a whole-grain alternative (whole wheat flour, oat flour, etc.). The key here is to have fun with this process remembering that most cravings can be satisfied in a healthier way.

STEP 4: Clean out your pantry

This is important because it is harder to succumb to temptation if it is not staring you in the face day after day. So, roll up your sleeves and dig in; toss out all of your processed, refined, oil-laden products and replacing them with healthy alternatives. We have included a sample list of pantry essentials to help guide you (see Appendix G).

STEP 5: Identify quick and easy favorites

Specifically, three or four meals (pasta, stir "fry," soups, etc.), three or four snacks (pita and humus, chips and salsa, fruit, etc.), and several sauces (peanut, cashew cheese, etc.) that you love and can easily prepare. The key is to become adept at preparing these base dishes. Have these ingredients available to you at all times. Meals or snacks that need to be prepared can be made ahead of time and kept in the freezer. It is important to plan ahead so that you can have this convenience when you need it.

STEP 6: Commit to this program for one month.

By commit, we mean give it 100% of your effort. Keep in mind that the larger the leap you take (meaning the closer you get to an A+ on the Food Continuum[34]) the greater the benefit you will reap. For those of you interested in just getting your feet wet, consider adding fruits and vegetables while limiting/eliminating animal products, oils, and refined foods. For those of you wishing to dive in, make whole plant foods the basis of your diet and eliminate animal products, oil, and refined foods altogether. No matter what you decide, find your comfort zone and begin your journey. If you get lost on your way or just need additional support, we will be happy to help motivate, encourage, and help you find your way.

If followed correctly, the Exsalus Health Program
can help you lose weight, decrease your cholesterol,
stabilize your blood sugar, lower your blood pressure,
improve your bowel function, revitalize your energy,
as well as

help prevent, slow down, eliminate, or reverse the following: acne, allergies, arthritis, asthma, autoimmune disease (lupus, ankylosing spondylitis, multiple sclerosis, etc.), cancer, chronic fatigue, constipation, dementia, depression, diabetes, diarrhea, heart disease, high blood pressure, high cholesterol, gastrointestinal disorders (including reflux), gout, headaches, impotence, inflammatory bowel disease, insomnia, irritable bowel syndrome, obesity, and rheumatoid arthritis, among other things.

After one month of following the program, your success will be the factor that keeps you motivated to continue. At this point, you can assess your progress and determine whether you are comfortable where you are or decide you are ready to take it to the next level on the Food Continuum[34] and Optimum Health Continuum. In this manner, you can continue to tweak your program to suit your needs and meet your goals.

And always remember the basics: "Keep It Simple & Keep It Whole" (meaning low-fat, plant-based, and whole foods).

You can cook it, bake it, or eat it raw
as long as you are making whole plant foods
the base of your diet.

This is the key: don't allow yourself to get bogged down in the minutia, as this will become extremely overwhelming. For example, does it really matter whether you cook your broccoli or eat it raw? Cooking broccoli could be argued either way: cooking broccoli might deplete some of the nutrients versus cooking broccoli makes some of the nutrients more available. The bottom line is, eat the broccoli; we have yet to see a patient who is sick because they ate too much cooked broccoli instead of raw broccoli. As another example, why debate whether MSG is healthy or not when MSG is generally found in unhealthy foods. The take-home message then becomes, if you "Keep It Simple & Keep It Whole" you will avoid the MSG debate (and others like it) in the first place.

For those of you who are tired of the status quo, you owe it to yourselves and to those who love you to give this plan a shot. The worst thing that could happen is that you do not experience any change and you return to your previous lifestyle – no harm no foul. But, the best that can happen is that you regain your health and your vitality so that you can enjoy the long and happy life you so deserve.

One last thing:

Remember that slips may happen,
and if they do, see them as learning opportunities,

because it is more important that you focus on what you can do differently next time rather than get upset and punish yourself. Really, the only way to fail is to stop trying. We know that this diet can be delicious and can help you feel fantastic. We wouldn't be living our plan or recommending it to you otherwise. But like we discussed earlier, this process will be like learning a new language. As such, chances are you will fumble before you are fluent but that does not mean you are failing. We know, as we have been through the process and paid our dues in time and effort to become fluent in this language of optimum health. That is why

we are certain that with continued practice and
a healthy dose of desire, you will become fluent as well.

Take-home messages:

- **Steps for success:**
  - o **Identify your objectives and set realistic goals for your transition.**
  - o **Develop a palatable and satisfying meal plan.**
  - o **Remember you can do this around any schedule (including traveling and eating out).**
  - o **Keep a food diary.**
  - o **Clean out your pantry.**
  - o **Commit to this program for one month.**
- **See any slip-ups as learning opportunities, because the only way to fail is to stop trying!**
- **"Keep It Simple & Keep It Whole."**

"Let food be thy medicine and let thy medicine be thy food."
—Hippocrates

Appendix A: Optimum Health Continuum

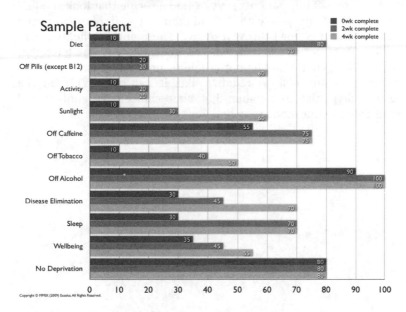

This is a sample of the Optimum Health Continuum (OHC) we use to evaluate our patients' progress. As you can see, optimum health is comprehensive and incorporates many aspects of our lives, including our diet, state of physical health, habits, and overall well-being. The idea is to continue to move to the right (i.e., towards 100%). The key, however, is to do so without significantly compromising satiation, satisfaction, or well-being. In other words, you cannot be hungry, frustrated, or deprived. You can achieve this by finding your individual balance so that this new diet and lifestyle remains delicious and fun. For example, in the "Diet" section you want to always remember nutrients (i.e., your whole foods: fruits, vegetables, including the starchy ones, whole grains, and legumes) first, but you do not want to limit yourself to only raw or steamed vegetables and brown rice. Although this may move your diet portion of the OHC way over to the right, you will most likely experience deprivation that will result in a decline in overall well-being. This is NOT optimal health and more often than not marks the beginning of a downward spiral resulting in discontinuation of the program. So instead, make a lasagna or Thai peanut noodles, have the peanut/cashew/pesto sauces available to you, allow yourself to indulge in treats from time to time (including carrot cake and chocolate brownies) (see recipes in Appendix I). In essence, broaden your menu choices so that you do not feel limited or deprived. Address your cravings, and remember that there is a way to modify virtually any recipe to a healthier version; don't be afraid to challenge yourself and experiment with the options. As one of our patients says, "I find a recipe that looks good, I tweak it to meet my dietary needs, and then I try it. If it is good I keep the recipe and if is not I throw it away." The point is, when you are experimenting, not every dish will be gourmet; but don't let that reflect on the general diet as not edible or not tasty. Instead, realize that this was one dish you didn't like; it happens EVEN on the American diet. Also, remember that your choices are endless and limited only by your motivation and your creativity.

Appendix B: Food Continuum[34] and 3-Phase Eating

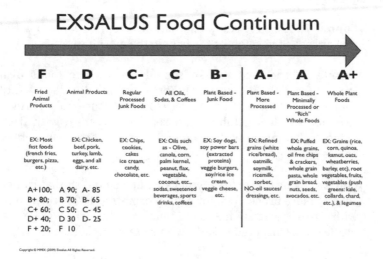

EXSALUS Food Continuum

F	D	C-	C	B-	A-	A	A+
Fried Animal Products	Animal Products	Regular Processed Junk Foods	All Oils, Sodas, & Coffees	Plant Based - Junk Food	Plant Based - More Processed	Plant Based - Minimally Processed or "Rich" Whole Foods	Whole Plant Foods
EX: Most fast foods (french fries, burgers, pizza, etc.)	EX: Chicken, beef, pork, turkey, lamb, eggs, and all dairy, etc.	EX: Chips, cookies, cakes ice cream, candy, chocolate, etc.	EX: Oils such as - Olive, canola, corn, palm kernel, peanut, flax, vegetable, coconut, etc., sodas, sweetened beverages, sports drinks, coffees	EX: Soy dogs, soy power bars (extracted proteins) veggie burgers, soy/rice ice cream, veggie cheese, etc.	EX: Refined grains (white rice/bread), oatmilk, soymilk, ricemilk, sorbet, NO-oil sauces/ dressings, etc.	EX: Puffed whole grains, oil free chips & crackers, whole grain pasta, whole grain bread, nuts, seeds, avocados, etc.	EX: Grains (rice, corn, quinoa, kamut, oats, wheatberries, barley, etc), root vegetables, fruits, greens: kale, collards, chard, etc.), & legumes

A+100; A 90; A- 85
B+ 80; B 70; B- 65
C+ 60; C 50; C- 45
D+ 40; D 30 D- 25
F + 20; F 10

This Food Continuum[34] is intended to serve as a guide to help you categorize your overall diet, a new food pyramid if you will. The idea is to try and live to the right of the vertical black line (the A-, A, and A+ zones). Specifically, when you sit down for a meal, you want to eat the most nutritious foods first (i.e., those from the A+ category). Then, you want to move down the continuum (to the left) to the A, A- foods. We often think of it as using the A and A- foods to season the A+ foods. In this manner, you insure that you will 1) get your nutrients in, and 2) fill up on the more nutritious foods before moving on to the less nutritious ones.

Here are a few sample meals demonstrating how to move along the Food Continuum[34]:

1) Begin with raw or cooked vegetables that you can dip into a tasty sauce; next have some Thai peanut noodles and steamed vegetable dumplings; next have a piece of fruit; and finally have a small piece of carrot cake.
2) Begin with a quinoa salad; next have some lentil loaf with mashed potatoes; next have a chilled mango; and, finally, enjoy a few truffles.

For those of you trying to lose weight, this notion of eating down the Food Continuum[34] is extremely important. You may want to break down your meal into 3 courses (also known as 3-Phase Eating):

3-Phase Eating

> **Course 1:** The first course should always be a large bowl of raw or cooked vegetables (or fruit in the morning).
>
> **Course 2:** The next course should be a whole foods dish (comes from the A+ section). Some examples include: lentil soup over brown rice, brown rice/beans/lettuce/salsa, brown rice sushi with vegetables and seaweed, oatmeal with fruit, quinoa salad mixed with cranberries and assorted vegetables, and so on.
>
> **Course 3:** For this course, you can add a side dish that can be slightly more processed. For example, oil-free 100% corn chips with salsa, lasagna, macaroni and cashew "cheese," pizza, whole grain/sprouted breads, whole grain crackers, etc.

Remember that you want to make the majority of the meal consist of course 1 (your "weight loss medicine and multivitamin") and course 2 (your "filler") and supplement those two with course 3 (optional).

Finally, for dessert start with fruit whenever possible. Try picking exciting and sweet-tasting fruits like chilled mangos, frozen bananas (which taste like ice cream), frozen grapes, melons, etc. There will be some days where this will be satisfying enough. On those other days when you are craving more, still have the fruit first and then have the more processed and calorie-dense desserts.

Appendix C: Calorie Density and Eating Whole

A whole food like brown rice has 500 calories per pound, but if you process it into a whole-grain flour (by removing water and finely chopping it up) then it becomes 1500 calories per pound. This is the concept of calorie density. Caloric density is basically the amount of calories you can pack into a given amount of food. Processed foods are more calorie dense because they are lacking much of the water and fiber (which contributes bulk but no calories) found in whole foods. In other words, by removing the fiber and water the food becomes much more concentrated and therefore higher in calories and lower in bulk (see Calorie Density Table below for more examples). This does not necessarily make processed foods a bad thing; it should, however, make us more conscientious when we are consuming processed foods (especially if we are trying to lose weight).

Calorie Density Table

WHOLE FOODS	CALORIES per POUND		MORE PROCESSED FOODS	CALORIES per POUND
Cabbage	100	→	Fast Food Coleslaw	700
Tomatoes	150	→	Sun Dried Tomatoes	1150
Apricots	200	→	Dried Apricots	1100
Grapes	300	→	Raisins	1350
Bananas	400	→	Banana Chips	2350
Sweet Potato	400	→	Sweet Potato Fries	1100
Brown Rice	500	→	Brown Rice Flour	1500
Corn	500	→	Chips with Oil	2500
Olives	600	→	Olive Oil	4000
Avocado	750	→	Avocado Oil	4000

and others:

FOODS	CALORIES PER POUND
Lentils	500
Black Beans	600
Pure Sugar	1800
Chocolate	2200
Seeds	2650
Nuts	2800

As you can see, the whole foods on the left naturally have a lower caloric density than the more processed foods on the right. The exceptions being nuts and seeds, which is why we tell you to use them sparingly or as a "seasoning."

The take-home message is:

- **Processing foods increases their caloric density.**

- **Processed does not necessarily mean unhealthy (be careful here though because many, if not most, processed foods are indeed unhealthy).**

- **Even healthy processed foods are NOT as healthy as whole foods.**

- **"Keep it Simple and Keep it Whole" whenever possible.**

Appendix D: Identifying Challenges and Planning Ahead

This page is intended to help you identify your obstacles/rate-limiting steps and come up with strategies to help you better prepare for and thereby manage these challenges. Please take the time to fill this chart in so that you can be prepared for any obstacles that could potentially lie between you and your success (see Chapter 14 for more details).

Identifying Your Challenges Worksheet

Rate-limiting step	Strategy 1	Strategy 2	Strategy 3
Ex. No time for cooking	Find one or two evenings or a weekend day and make several dishes that you can refrigerate and freeze for the week.	Create a buddy system with friends/co-workers and share the cooking. For example, take turns with four other co-workers so that each member is responsible for bringing five servings of a healthy lunch one day a week. This way you only have to make one lunch a week.	Find restaurants willing to accommodate your dietary needs and buy meals from them.
#1			
#2			

Appendix E: Meal Planning

We have found that planning is one of the key steps to a successful transition to health. As such, we have included a meal plan calendar for you to fill out on a weekly basis.

The purpose of the meal plan is several-fold:

1) It aids in organizing your meals for the week. You can even put a shopping list on the back so that you know exactly what foods you need to buy that week. By creating this global picture, you can better balance your meals to make sure you are getting plenty of the A+ foods without depriving yourself too much (i.e., making sure to add in the side dishes and occasional desserts);

2) It makes shopping easier because by knowing what your meals will be, you can do one big shopping spree for the week; and

3) It helps to hold you accountable for what you will be consuming for the week, making you less likely to become overwhelmed at any given moment and succumb to less healthy or unhealthy choices.

The following are some steps and strategies to help you in creating your meal plans and preparing your meals:

1) Organize your meals for the week. Choose a variety of foods, making sure that they are starch-based and that some of the weekly foods are rich enough to prevent a sense of deprivation. Remember that you CANNOT live off of vegetables for ALL meals ALL week long; you MUST include starches (root vegetables, whole grains, and legumes) and/or fruits with most, if not every, meal.

2) Develop a shopping list for the week based on the meal calendar you created. This will make shopping easier because you can get it all done in one shot. Also, this helps with food preparation because you will know in advance that you have the ingredients at home ready for you to make your meals. You can even save your weekly meal plans so that over time you accumulate different weeks worth of meals and the corresponding shopping lists. After the first 4-6 weeks you can start rotating through the old ones rather than having to come up with new ones.

3) You can decide to cook all your meals on one day, (maybe a weekend day) and then freeze them (this is an especially good

idea for people who know they will be busy during the week), or choose a few days during the week to make your meals.

4) You can make extra for dinner and then have leftovers for lunch.

5) You can partner with a buddy to develop a meal plan and then break up the cooking responsibilities. Another option is to make one person "the shopper" and another "the cook" for the week and then switch roles. There are many options, so choose the one that works best for you.

6) Make sure to include any plans for dining out (if you know where you are going and what you will be having you can write that in, otherwise fill it in after the meal).

Meal Plan Calendar

	Mon	Tues	Wed	Thur	Fri	Sat	Sun
Breakfast							
Snack							
Lunch							
Snack							
Dinner							
Snack							

Appendix F: Food Diary

For those of you interested in monitoring your progress, keeping a Food Diary will prove very helpful. To be an effective tool, however, the Food Diary MUST include EVERYTHING you put in your mouth: every taste, nibble, bite, etc. In this manner, if you are not achieving the results you desire, you can look back and assess why that might be happening. And if you continue to struggle, we would be happy to see you in our private practice (or via a phone education session) and work with you personally to further explore and help explain the reasons for the inconsistencies (you can reach us at info@Exsalus.com).

From our experience, whenever our patients come to us frustrated and discouraged that this "diet and lifestyle doesn't work," 100% of the time it is because of a misunderstanding that has resulted in not complying (often unknowingly) with the program. Even more specifically, and more often than not, the confusion stems from not completely understanding how to apply the Food Continuum[34] to daily meals or how to incorporate the 3-Phase Eating Plan (see Appendix B).

This is an extremely important concept and a key ingredient to your success, so we highly recommend that you spend some time familiarizing yourself with the Food Continuum[34], 3-Phase Eating Plan, and the practical examples given in Appendix B.

Appendix F: Food Diary

DATE:		Note which foods fulfilled which phases:	3-Phase Eating
AM meal COURSE 1:	AM meal COURSE 2:	AM meal COURSE 3: (optional)	COURSE 1 = 1st BOWL of food *(NOT optional)*
			"Multivitamin" or "Weight-Loss Medicine"
			Veggies - ideally RAW but can be cooked (ideally something green and leafy like kale, spinach, broccoli, etc.)
Snack & Comments:			**Note**: For Breakfast, high water content WHOLE fruits OK but try to add greens (ex: green smoothie)
Noon meal COURSE 1:	Noon meal COURSE 2:	Noon meal COURSE 3: (optional)	COURSE 2 = 2nd BOWL of food *(NOT optional)*
			"FILLER" or "Meat of the Meal"
			WHOLE Starches - Sweet Potatoes, Squash, Oats, Quinoa, Brown Rice, Corn, Lentils, Beans, Potatoes, Wheat Berries, Bulgur, Barley, Buckwheat, etc.
			Can eat more than one bowl of phase 2 if you like
Snacks & Comments:			COURSE 3 = 3rd BOWL of food *(optional)*
			"Flavor" or "Emotional Eating"
PM meal COURSE 1:	PM meal COURSE 2:	PM meal COURSE 3: (optional)	Slightly Processed Starches: corn tortillas, whole grain breads, oil-free chips, puffed grains, whole grain lasagna, whole grain pastas/noodles, burritos, enchiladas, quiche, veggie pizza, corn bread, etc.
			Avoid more refined foods (white flour/breads/pastas)
			Desserts *(optional)*
			Always have **WHOLE fruit first** then have richer OIL-FREE dessert
			Nuts, Seeds, Avocados, Olives, Soy, etc. (richer plant foods) *(optional)*
Snacks & Comments:			Use as a **"Seasoning"** in/on your meal ONLY (if used at all - careful if weight loss is your goal)

Appendix G: Pantry Essentials

Remember to read product labels to make sure that there is no oil added to your pantry essentials.

Grains (brown rice, barley, couscous)
Canned beans (pinto, kidney, garbanzo, black, fat-free refried, etc.)
Canned vegetables (corn, peas, carrots, artichokes, etc.)
Pasta (whole wheat, rice, quinoa)
Pizza crust – Nature's Highlights
Vegetable broth
Tomato sauce and paste
Dr. Mc Dougall's Right Foods Smart Cups (travel soup, oatmeal)
Bottled salsa
Low-sodium soy sauce
Date sugar
Other sweeteners if needed (maple syrup, honey, brown sugar, etc.)
Tabasco sauce (or other hot sauce)
Dip and dressing mixes (Simply Organic)
Fat-free salad dressings –assorted (Honey Mustard, Italian, French)
Condiments: mustard, ketchup, barbeque sauces, etc.
Vinegars: rice vinegar, wine vinegar, apple cider vinegar, etc.
Cornstarch or arrowroot
Ener-G Egg Replacer
Wonderslim Cocoa Powder (fat-free)
Whole-wheat flour
Soy, rice, or oat milk
Oats (rolled, steel cut, etc.)
Raisins
Herbal teas
Coffee substitutes (Teeccino)
Potatoes, onions, and garlic
Baked tortilla chips (no oil) – La Reina
Puffed grain cereals
Brown rice cakes
Air-popped popcorn (no oil)
Spices (basil, oregano, onion powder, garlic powder, ginger, crushed black pepper, dill weed, nutmeg, cinnamon, curry powder, paprika, cayenne, turmeric). Note: check for and avoid additives like sugar and preservatives.

Appendix H: Cooking without Oil

Here are some oil alternatives to use in cooking and baking.

365 - Applesauce

Annie Chun's – Soy Ginger, Korean Barbeque Sauce

Annie's Naturals - Worcestershire sauce, Shiitake Mushroom Sauce, Teriyaki Sauce

Ayla's Organics - Cajun, Curry, Szechwan, Thai Sauce

Cindy's Kitchen – All Natural Sun-dried Tomato Fat-Free Dressing Marinade

Libby's – 100% Pure Canned Pumpkin

McIhenny Co. - Tabasco Sauce

Nabisco Brands - A1 Steak Sauce

Nakano USA - Seasoned Rice Vinegar

Newman's Own – Balsamic Vinegar

Robbie's – BBQ Sauce

S & D Foods, Inc. - Parrot Brand Enchilada Sauce

Thai Kitchen – Sweet Red Chili

Trader Joe's - Organic Unsweetened Applesauce

Appendix I: Recipes

How to sauté without oil (onions, for example):

1) Use a good non-stick pan (we like the cookware by Berndes or Swiss Diamond) and let it get hot.

2) To the hot, dry pan add your chopped onion and allow it to start to brown. It may appear to stick a little but let it get brown and caramelize without adding any water (otherwise you will start poaching the onion instead of sautéing it).

3) Once it starts to get brown add a couple of tablespoons of non-oil liquid (water, juice, broth, etc.) but not too much, as you don't want to cool the pan. The water added will bubble and steam.

4) Immediately mix the onions around the pan with a non-metal spatula, using the small amount of water just added to collect the brown, caramelized contents from the sides of the pan. The pan will have cooled from adding the water but will quickly heat up again as the onions continue to darken and caramelize further.

5) Add another couple of tablespoons of water to the pan and repeat the same process again until the onions are brown and caramelized.

NOTE: The key to this process is that you need to periodically add liquid (in small amounts) compared to oil which you only had to add once.

Ideas for snacks:
- Assorted vegetables dipped in fat-free and oil-free hummus (e.g., Oasis brand)
- Oil-free corn chips (ex. La Reina) and guacamole or hummus (see #1)
- Apple with a tablespoon of almond butter or peanut butter
- Assorted vegetables or corn chips (see #2) dipped in bean dip
- 365 Woven Wheats dipped in cashew "cheese," artichoke, and spinach dip
- Fruit

Breakfast

Crockpot Hot Cereal
(thank you Mona Howard)

½ cup any grain (rolled oats, barley, etc.)
½ cup steel cut oats
½ cup chopped dates
½ tsp salt
4½ cups water
½ tsp vanilla or almond extract
¼ tsp cinnamon
1½ cups berries

1. Put grains, dates, salt, and water in a crockpot.
2. Turn the heat to low, and cook overnight, or for 6-8 hours.
3. When ready to serve, stir in vanilla or almond extract, cinnamon, and berries

✳

Honey Please Do! Smoothie

1 whole honey dew melon chilled
6 oz bag of spinach
2 bananas (frozen)
1 cup blueberries (frozen)
1-2 tbsp ground flax seeds (optional)

1. Take a whole honey dew melon and scrape (just the insides) into a blender.
2. Add spinach and blend.
3. Add 1½ -2 frozen bananas and about 1 cup of frozen blueberries and blend.
4. Add ground flax seed (1-2 tbsp) if you like.

❋

Maple-Pecan French Toast
(thank you Davida Becker and Gil Pulde)

¾ cup chopped pecans, toasted
1¼ cup soy milk or other dairy-free milk
4 oz. soft silken tofu, drained
1 tsp pure vanilla extract
¾ cup pure maple syrup
8 slices whole-grain or sprouted bread

1. Place ¼ cup of the pecans in a blender and grind into a powder. Add the soy milk, tofu, vanilla and ¼ cup of the maple syrup and process until smooth.
2 Pour into a large, shallow bowl and dip in the bread, coating both sides evenly with the batter.
3. Preheat the oven to 200 degrees F. Heat a non-stick griddle or large skillet over medium heat. Add the prepared bread in batches and cook until browned on both sides, 4-5 minutes total. Keep the cooked French toast warm in the oven while you prepare the remaining slices.
4. In a small saucepan, combine the remaining ½ cup maple syrup and the remaining ½ cup pecans and heat until warm. Spoon over the French toast and serve at once.

*

Morning Smoothie

1-2 cups of non-dairy milk, juice, and/or some other combination
(add more or less depending on how sweet, creamy, and thick you like
your smoothie)
6-12 oz of spinach (can substitute or add other greens)
¾ cup strawberries
¾ cup blueberries
¾ cup cherries
1 frozen banana
¾ cup seedless grapes
½ cup walnuts
1-2 tbsp ground flax seed

1. Blend spinach and soymilk into liquid.
2. Add fruit. Note, use some or all frozen fruit to make smoothie
thicker OR use fresh fruit along with some ice. Substitute any fruits
above with fruits you prefer (for example, mango would be delicious).
You also can just use one or two fruits (for example, bananas and
mango taste delicious with spinach).
3. Be sure to add greens, as it is a great way to incorporate fresh raw
vegetables.

*

Oatmeal

2 cups oatmeal
6 cups fluids (we use 5 cups of water and 1 cup of apple juice but you
may adjust as necessary to taste; to make sweeter add more apple
juice and less water)

1. Put all ingredients into a pot, bring to a boil and simmer for about
10-20 minutes until desired consistency.
2. Serve warm or cold...Delicious!!!
3. Toppings may include cinnamon, apples, bananas, and raisins.

Sauces and Salad Dressings

Berry Salad Dressing
(thank you Mona Howard)

1 pound berries
3 tbsp white balsamic vinegar
Coarsely ground white pepper

1. Blend and serve.

❋

Orange-Ginger-Sesame Salad Dressing
(thank you Mona Howard)

½ cup seasoned rice vinegar
½ cup orange juice
½ tsp grated peeled fresh ginger (remember, you can keep grated ginger root in the freezer to use when needed)
½-1 tsp soy sauce (adjust to taste)
1-2 tsp sesame seeds

1. Blend and serve.

*

Peanut Sauce

Can be used as dressing on salads/vegetables or mixed in pasta/noodle dish.

In sauce pan add:
4 tbsp of 100% peanut butter
½ cup soy sauce
½ cup seasoned rice wine vinegar
½ cup sugar (we use date sugar)
2 cups water
¾ tsp dried cilantro
¾ tsp dried basil
½ tsp dried garlic
½ tsp dried ginger

1. Blend all ingredients together with whisk on medium-high heat (add more water if too strong).
2. If using regular sugar, add 4 tbsp of thickening agent (corn starch or arrowroot) completely dissolved in 3-4 tbsp of water. Using a whisk, blend starch liquid into sauce mixture while on heat (use more or less starch depending on how thick you like it).

NOTE: If using date sugar skip step 2 (because date sugar will naturally thicken the mixture and taste delicious!).

Side Dishes

Hummus
(thank you Shoshana Pulde)

30 oz can of garbanzo beans
4 cloves of garlic
juice of half a lemon
1 tbsp tahini
salt and pepper to taste

1. Put all ingredients in food processor or blender and process until smooth.
2. Keep covered and refrigerated.

✴

Eggplant Dip
(thank you Shoshana Pulde)

5 large eggplants
5 cloves of garlic crushed
juice of 1 large lemon
1-2 tbsp tahini
5 green onions chopped
salt and pepper to taste (about 1 tsp salt and a dash of pepper)

1. Roast whole eggplants in oven (or on barbecue) at 400 degrees for about 40-50 minutes (until soft).
2. Remove from oven and let eggplants cool.
3. Scoop inside of eggplant into a bowl and mash, discard the peels.
4. Let stand for about 30 minutes and discard any accumulated juices.
5. Add crushed garlic, lemon juice, tahini, green onions, and salt and pepper and mix together.
6. Keep covered and refrigerated.

✴

Low-fat Guacamole
(thank you Mona Howard)

1 can (15 oz) white kidney beans (cannelloni), rinsed and drained
1 ripe avocado
1 jar salsa (mild, moderate, or spicy)
lime juice, garlic powder, black pepper

1. Mash the beans in a food processor with some fresh squeezed lime juice and puree until smooth (lemon juice works just as well).
2. Mash the avocado with a fork or potato masher and add to the bean mixture.
3. Add salsa of choice to desired consistency/taste.
4. Add sprinkle of garlic powder and some pepper to taste.

Note: if you choose not to use salsa from a jar then chop tomatoes, onions, jalapenos, and some cilantro. Some people always add extra cilantro to jarred salsa anyway so experiment. The bottom line is to use the beans as a substitute for the avocado.

❋

Roasted Beet Salad with Toasted Walnuts
(thank you Chef Leslie McKenna)

6 beets, greens removed and washed and chopped
2 large red onions cut into 1-inch slices
1 tbsp dried basil leaves
4 large basil leaves, chiffonade (plus additional for garnish)
½ cup walnuts, toasted and chopped
1 shallot, minced
1 clove garlic, minced
3 tbsp almond butter or peanut butter
1 tbsp warm water
2 tbsp balsamic vinegar
1 cup extra firm or baked tofu (optional)
salt and pepper to taste

For Dressing:
1. Combine the shallots, garlic, chopped basil, almond butter, balsamic, reserved beet juice, salt and pepper and mix well.
2. Add warm water if dressing is too thick, otherwise omit.
3. Season with salt and pepper. Set aside.

For Salad:
1. Preheat oven to 400 degrees.
2. Wrap the beets in foil and place on a baking sheet and bake for 1 hour or until soft. Open the foil but leave the beets in the foil to catch all of the juices. Make sure you reserve all the juices from the beets for the dressing. Set aside.
3. Slice the onions and season with salt, pepper and dried basil.
4. Heat the grill pan (preferably non-stick) until smoking hot and spray a paper towel with water and lightly rub onto the grill.
5. Place onion slices on grill and turn down heat to medium. Let them cook for 4 minutes or until they are scored with a nice grill mark and carefully flip them over and cook for another 4 to 5 minutes until they are soft. Remove to a plate and let cool, then rough chop them and add them to a bowl.
6. Once the beets are cool, using a paper towel, gently remove the skin and chop into a large dice, and add to the onions.
7. Place a little water into a pan and add the chopped beet greens, and steam cover until wilted. Drain well and season with salt and pepper. Roughly chop and add to the beets.
8. Add the toasted walnuts.

❋

Tabouleh
(thank you Shoshana Pulde)

1 cup bulgur wheat (preferably thin or fine grain)
1 cup hot water
5 green onions chopped
2 cloves garlic minced
2 Persian cucumbers diced
2 large tomatoes diced
½ cup parsley chopped
juice of 1 lemon
salt and pepper to taste (½ tsp each approximately)

1. Combine bulgur and water.
2. Cover and let stand for about 30 minutes.
3. Fluff bulgur.
4. Add all ingredients and mix.
5. Keep covered and refrigerated.

Soups

Cabbage Potato Stew
(thank you Mona Howard)

2 cups veggie broth
4 large potatoes cut into large pieces
1 head cabbage, sliced into strips
Salt, pepper, dill weed (or caraway seeds) to taste

1. Lightly sauté the cabbage in a small amount of broth.
2. Add potatoes with remainder of broth and simmer.
3. Keep covered until potatoes are tender.
4. You can add more broth to make more of a soup or let it thicken like a stew.

Note: Works well as a hearty side dish or can be used as an entrée. Very versatile.

*

Cauliflower and Pea Soup
(thank you Shoshana Pulde)

Sauté 1 tbsp flour or corn starch until it becomes an off-white color.
Add enough water to just cover the flour and mix so the flour doesn't clump together.
Add 2 heads of cauliflower (washed and separated into florets)
Add 1-2 cups of green peas (fresh or frozen)
Add vegetable broth to cover vegetables
Cook until vegetables are soft (about 25-30minutes)
Add ½ cup of chopped dill
Season with salt and pepper to taste

Note: If you like your peas crunchier add them 20-25 minutes into the cooking.

*

Dr. Lederman's Black Bean Soup

In a big pot add all ingredients:
1 cup carrots
1 cup celery
1 cup onion
6 cans black beans (14.5 ounce cans)
1 lb frozen corn
4 cans of crushed tomatoes spiced with green chilies
2 banana peppers chopped up
1 jalapeno pepper chopped up

Cook in pot until boils and then simmer for 30 minutes.

While soup is cooking: Cook in pan (sauté with vegetable broth or water) for about 10 minutes.
½ cup onions
1 head kale
1 head collards
1 head chard

1. Put cooked greens and ½ -1 cup of fresh cilantro in a food processor (until blended).
2. Mix blended greens with soup until stirred in completely.
3. Serve in a bowl and mix with crushed oil-free, tortilla chips.

＊

Hearty Dal Soup
(thank you Mary McDougall)

3¼ cups water
1 onion, chopped
2 cloves garlic, crushed
1½ tsp grated fresh ginger
1 tsp smoked paprika (must use smoked)
¼ tsp ground cumin
freshly ground black pepper
1 cup red lentils
1 15 ounce can garbanzos, drained and rinsed
1 14½ ounce can diced tomatoes
2 cups chunked sweet potatoes
1 tbsp lemon juice
1-2 tsp chili paste (Sambal Oelek)
2-4 cups fresh chopped chard

1. Place ¼ cup of the water in a large soup pot.
2. Add the onion and garlic.
3. Cook, stirring occasionally for 3-4 minutes, until softened.
4. Add the ginger, paprika, cumin and several twists of freshly ground pepper.
5. Mix in well, then add the remaining water, the lentils, garbanzos, tomatoes and potatoes.
6. Bring to a boil, reduce heat, cover and simmer for 50 minutes, until lentils are tender.
7. Add lemon juice, chili paste (start with 1 tsp and add more to taste) and chard.
8. Cook for an additional 5-7 minutes, until chard is tender.
9. Season with a bit of sea salt, if desired.
10. Serve hot.

❃

Split Pea Soup
(thank you Shoshana Pulde)

1 onion – chopped
1½ cups split peas
2 large carrots – shredded
10 cups boiling water
2 tbsp chicken soup style vegetable powder (vegan)

1. Sauté onion until yellow, add split peas and carrots and mix.
2. Boil water and add chicken soup vegetable powder (note: can use vegetable broth instead of the water and soup powder)
3. Cook on low heat about an hour, mix periodically so it does not stick.
4. Add salt and pepper to taste, decorate with chopped parsley.

❃

Ellen Neufeld's Miso Soup
(thank you Ellen Neufeld)

7-8 cups water
1 tsp chopped garlic
3-4 sliced carrots
2 stalks sliced celery
½ package mushrooms sliced (heaping cup)
1 cup shelled frozen edamame
3 large stalks of bok choy (or chard) (stalks and leaves) chopped
4 oz. of half-cooked buckwheat soba noodles
Miso paste (dark miso, about 1/3 cup +/- another tbsp, or light miso ½ cup)
Soy sauce to taste

Bring 7-8 cups water to a boil and add garlic, sliced carrots, and celery, and boil until vegetables are tender. Add mushrooms and edamame and continue to boil until mushrooms are tender. Add bok choy (stalks and leaves), until bok choy is tender, then turn off flame. Take the half-cooked buckwheat soba noodles, drain, and run cold water over them; set aside. Dissolve miso paste in 4 ladles of soup broth in a separate bowl then add back to pot (adjust for desired taste). Add buckwheat noodles and soy sauce to taste (if using light miso). Optional: may also add cubed tofu with miso.

*

Mark Neufeld's Vegetable Soup
(thank you Mark Neufeld)

3 boxes vegetable broth
2 large sweet potatoes washed and unpeeled
1 lb carrots washed and unpeeled
1 large parsnip washed and unpeeled
1 large turnip washed and unpeeled
1 red potato washed and unpeeled
1 leek
1 large yellow onion
½ bunch fresh dill
½ bunch fresh parsley
½ bunch fresh basil
2 large handfuls raw spinach
Garlic powder to taste
Salt and pepper to taste

Roughly cut all vegetables and herbs, and place into a soup pot with the broth, garlic powder, salt and pepper. Boil vegetables until soft. Strain broth into the pot, and put the vegetables into a blender; puree and pour mixture back into the pot with the broth. Next, peel, chop and put into soup mixture:

1 lb carrots
2 sweet potatoes
1 package of sliced mushrooms
½ bunch green onions, diced
1 yellow onion, diced
½ bunch fresh parsley, chopped
½ bunch fresh dill, chopped
½ bunch fresh basil, chopped

Simmer until the vegetables are soft, and serve.

✳

Mom's Miso
(thank you Mom)

¼ cup vegetable broth
2 leeks (white part only, well rinsed, and sliced)
2 cloves garlic
1 bunch chard (or Bok Choy), chopped, (aprox. ½ pound) separate leaves from stems and chop stems
4 medium carrots (aprox ¾ pound), chopped
4 ounces buckwheat noodles (soba)
1 cup edamame (fresh or frozen)
½ cup miso (can be found on shelf or in refrigerated section, once the shelf type is open, refrigerate.
2 ½ quarts water

1. Using veggie broth, sauté leeks and garlic, stirring occasionally
2. Add chard stems to pot and continue to cook until soft/tender, aprox 10 minutes
3. Add water to pot, increase heat and bring to boil.
   Add carrots and reduce heat to simmer until carrots are tender, approximately another 10 minutes
4. Bring a separate pot of water to boil to cook the soba noodles and cook till tender (3-4 minutes). Do not cook in soup pot because the noodles will absorb too much of the soup broth
5. Drain noodles and run under cold water and set aside
6. Add chopped chard leaves and edamame to soup and continue to cook until chard is wilted
7. Remove 1 cup of hot soup water and swirl the miso into this water; return the miso/water mixture to the soup pot. (note: I continued to add miso to the pot until it tasted the way I wanted it to taste. I think the amount of miso ultimately depends on the brand/type you buy.)
8. Add noodles and serve.

Entrees

Ethiopian Split Peas
(thank you Shoshana Pulde)

1 lb yellow split peas
3½ cups water, reserve ½ cup for later
1 large onion, diced
3 tbsp tomato paste
1-2 cloves garlic, pressed
½ tsp ground ginger OR one 1-inch-long piece fresh ginger (peeled and finely chopped)
½ tsp ground turmeric (optional)
½ tsp ground black pepper
salt to taste

1. Soak split peas for at least one hour. Then drain and rinse.
2. Sauté onion and garlic in enough water so they don't stick.
3. Add tomato paste.
4. Add 3 cups water, split peas and remaining spices.
5. Bring to a boil, then cover and simmer for about 35 minutes.
6. Check periodically and give it a stir. The water should evaporate, but if the peas start to stick, add more water and simmer again. You want the peas to be slightly chunky/slightly creamy.
7. Serve over brown rice or quinoa. (optional)

*

Lasagna
(thank you Mary McDougall)

This recipe is easier than it looks and you can make a lot and freeze the leftovers in separate squares.

Prepare the following before assembling the lasagna. Also preheat oven to 350 degrees and start boiling a large pot of water.

<u>Tofu Ricotta</u>:
1 12.3 ounce package silken tofu
1 lb fresh water-packed firm tofu
2 tsp minced garlic
¼ cup nutritional yeast
½ tsp salt
½ tsp pepper
1 tbsp parsley flakes
1 tsp basil
1 tsp oregano
¼ cup lemon juice
¼ cup soy milk (or other non-dairy milk)

Combine all of the above ingredients in a food processor and process until fairly smooth. Set aside.

In a pan sauté (with vegetable broth) the following:
1 onion chopped
1 16 oz package frozen chopped spinach (thaw and remove water or cook in pan until water cooks out)
1 Japanese eggplant chopped (optional)
1 box of mushrooms chopped
2 cups of tomatoes chopped
1 tbsp lemon juice
2 tsp garlic powder
2 tsp basil flakes
1 tsp of sweetener (raw sugar, agave, etc.)
1 tsp pepper
1-2 tsp salt to taste

Put cooked mixture in a bowl and set aside
Tomato sauce (can buy an oil-free sauce or do the following):
2 pounds of sweet grape or cherry tomatoes (or some other equivalent of sweet tomatoes) and blend in food processor
1-2 avocados blended with tomatoes (depends on desired creaminess)

2-3 cloves of garlic finely chopped
1 tbsp sweetener (raw sugar, agave, etc.)
1 tbsp Dijon mustard
1 tbsp of basil flakes
1 tbsp of oregano flakes

Blend all ingredients well in food processor

Lasagna:
1 recipe Tofu Ricotta
1 bowl of cooked vegetables
1 bowl of sauce
8 ounces lasagna noodles (try 100% brown rice lasagna noodles)
Parmesan cheese substitute

1. Bring a large pot of water to a boil.
2. Drop in the lasagna noodles, stir, and cook uncovered until just softened. Do not overcook.
3. Remove from water and drain, hanging them up to dry slightly OR use the no-boil lasagna noodles and eliminate this step entirely.
4. Put 1/3 of sauce on bottom of oblong baking dish and smooth over bottom.
5. Place 1 layer of the noodles over the sauce.
6. Then add half of the tofu mixture and smooth out.
7. Then spread half of the vegetable mixture.
8. Add another layer of noodles, the rest of the tofu mixture, the remaining vegetable mixture and the rest of the noodles.
9. Spoon the remaining sauce over the noodles (make sure you cover all the edges), sprinkle the Parmesan substitute over the top.
10. Cover with parchment paper and then cover with foil.
11. Bake for 60 minutes.
12. Remove from oven and let rest for 10 minutes before cutting.

Hints: This may be prepared ahead of time and refrigerated before baking. Add about 15 minutes to the baking time.

✳

Lentil and Pea Medley
(thank you Shoshana Pulde)

1 cup lentils
4 cloves garlic, minced
1 large red onion, diced
2 large onion, diced
6 celery stalks, sliced
½ medium red pepper, chopped
½ medium green pepper, chopped
½ medium orange pepper, chopped
½ medium yellow pepper, chopped
½ tsp ground turmeric
2 large tomatoes, peeled and chopped OR 14 oz can of diced tomatoes
1 cup frozen peas, thawed
1½ cups water OR fat-free vegetable broth
¼ cup cilantro (optional)
1 small jalapeno pepper (optional)

1. Sauté onions in water until golden brown.
2. Add all peppers, celery, and garlic and continue to sauté for about 10 minutes.
3. Rinse lentils and add them to mixture along with water (or vegetable broth) and turmeric.
4. Bring to a boil.
5. Reduce heat, cover, and simmer for about 20 minutes or until the lentils are soft.
6. Add in tomatoes, peas, and cilantro.
7. Continue to cook for about 5 more minutes.
8. Season with salt and black pepper to taste.
9. Serve over brown rice or quinoa. (optional)

*

Lentil Burgers
(thank you Shoshana Pulde)

1 cup dry red lentils, well rinsed
1½ cups rolled oats
2½ cups water
1 medium onion, diced
1 carrot, diced
½ tsp salt, 1 tsp black pepper
1 tbsp soy sauce

Barbeque sauce (optional):

1. Rinse the lentils in cold water until the water runs clear (this is a very important step).
2. Boil lentils in pot with water and salt for 20 minutes.
3. In a separate pan sauté onions in water until golden brown then add carrot and sauté for five more minutes.
4. Add this to the pot of lentils along with the black pepper, soy sauce, and oats.
5. While still warm, make patties.
6. Bake patties in oven at 375 degrees (for 20-30 minutes or until bottom is golden brown). Serve with barbeque sauce.

✵

Mac N "Cheese"
Cashew "Cheese" Sauce - can use as a versatile sauce, dip

1 cup raw cashews
1 cup water
1 tsp salt
1 tsp onion powder
¼ cup "Red Star" Nutritional Yeast
1 cup red onions
2-3 cups spinach (enough to make 1 cup cooked spinach)

in food processor add:
1. 1 cup raw cashews and blend into a powder
2. add ½ cup water and blend until creamy
3. add: salt, onion powder, "Red Star" Nutritional Yeast, ¼ cup water and blend all of the ingredients together until creamy
4. In a pan, sauté in water, 1 cup onions
5. Once onions are caramelized then add spinach and cover to steam. Add onion and spinach to above mixture and blend in processor until creamy. (add some water if too thick – should not need more than ¼ cup)
7. Can add chopped artichokes to make artichoke dip

Optional:
1. Mix cashew/onion/spinach mixture with 10-12 oz of cooked whole grain pasta (al dente). Spread evenly in a casserole dish. Bake at 350 degrees for 30 minutes.

*

Macaroni and Stuff

16 oz elbow macaroni, whole grain
1 small onion, chopped
2 garlic cloves, minced or 1 tsp of already minced garlic to taste
1½ cups water
15 oz can plain, oil-free tomato sauce (not pasta sauce)
10 oz frozen or canned corn
1 bag of frozen chopped spinach (or 5 cups fresh spinach or similar greens)
16 oz can pinto beans
3 tbsp nutritional yeast
4 tsp chili powder
½ tsp chipotle powder or more to taste
salt/pepper, hot sauce to taste
oil-free, baked corn chips

1. Boil pasta.
2. Sauté onion and garlic in small amount of veggie broth.
3. Add water, oil-free tomato sauce, corn, spinach, beans, yeast, and chili powder and mix completely until heated through.
4. Add all ingredients to cooked, drained pasta.
5. Simmer a bit and add more water if it is too dry.
6. Serve with broken tortilla chips on top.
7. Sprinkle hot sauce on top.

❋

Mushroom and Onion Casserole
(thank you Shoshana Pulde)

3 large onions, diced
2 lb white mushrooms, chopped
2 large potato, peeled and grated
¼ cup chopped dill
2 tomatoes, grated
1 tbsp nutritional yeast
¼ cup black pepper
salt to taste

1. Sauté onions in water until golden brown.
2. Add mushrooms and continue to sauté for 5-10 minutes.
3. Remove from stove.
4. Add potatoes, dill, tomatoes, nutritional yeast, pepper, and salt (optional).
5. Mix well and place in pan.
6. Bake at 350 degrees for about 45 minutes or until set.

❂

Potato and Veggie Casserole
(thank you Mona Howard)

4 cups veggie broth
1-2 garlic cloves
2 carrots, chopped
1 celery stalks, chopped
1 small onion, diced
1 cup green beans
1½ cups mushrooms (I prefer portabellas for a more hearty taste), sliced
1½ cup corn, fresh or frozen
½ tsp marjoram
¼ tsp sage
2 tsp Bragg's Liquid Aminos
2 tbsp cornstarch mixed with 1/3 cup cold water
4 large yukon gold potatoes, peeled (3-4 cups mashed)
salt, pepper to taste
¼ cup brewer's yeast, if desired

1. Place potatoes in a pot and boil until tender. Drain the potatoes and place in a bowl for later.
2. In a small amount of broth, sauté garlic, carrots, celery, and onion until softened.
3. Add remaining vegetables, spices, and broth and simmer until soft.
4. Blend the cornstarch or potato starch mixed with water and bring veggies to a boil, stirring until thickened. Place in casserole dish.
5. Mash the potatoes adding water or vegetable broth as needed to achieve desired consistency.
6. Season with salt and pepper.
7. Stir in ¼ cup nutritional yeast, if desired for a richer taste.
8. Spread potatoes on top of vegetables.
9. Sprinkle with paprika and bake at 350 for 30 minutes or until bubbling. You can briefly broil the top to crisp the potatoes

Note: extremely versatile, can use any combination of veggies. The addition of extra mushrooms seems to please the meat eater who is adjusting his palate.

＊

Rice Stuffed Tomatoes

6 large fresh tomatoes at room temperature
1½ cups of fresh sliced mushrooms
1 cup chopped onion
1 - 10 oz package of frozen, chopped spinach thawed and drained (can also use equivalent fresh)
2 medium avocados mashed
2 tsp minced garlic
1 tsp dried basil leaves, crushed
1 tsp brown sugar or agave nectar
½ tsp salt
¼ tsp ground black pepper
½ cup quick cooking rice
¼ cup plus 2 tbsp grated Vegan Parmesan cheese

1. Preheat oven to 400 degrees.
2. Use tomatoes that are fully ripe.
3. Cut a slice from the top of each tomato; remove pulp, leaving a ¼-inch thick shell; set aside.
4. Chop tomato pulp (makes about 3 ½ cups).
5. In a large skillet over high heat with some vegetable broth sauté mushrooms and onion; cook and stir until tender, about 10 minutes.
6. Add spinach, avocado, reserved chopped tomatoes, garlic, basil, sugar, salt and pepper.
7. Cook over low heat, stirring until flavors blend, about 10 minutes.
8. Stir in rice.
9. Remove from heat; cover and let stand for 5 minutes.
10. Stir in ¼ cup Vegan Parmesan cheese.
11. Place tomato shells in a 13 × 9 × 2-inch baking pan.
12. Spoon hot mixture into shells, dividing evenly.
13. Sprinkle 1 tsp Parmesan cheese on top of each.
14. Bake until tomatoes are hot and filling is golden, about 15 minutes.
15. Serve as a main dish.

❋

Stir-Fry (oil-free)

1 small red onion chopped
2 cloves of garlic chopped
1 tbsp fresh ginger grated finely
1-2 carrots shredded
1 cup fresh shitake mushrooms (can use dried if prefer but adjust quantity accordingly)
1 small Japanese eggplant cubed (optional)
½ - 1 cup of "Annie Chun's" soy ginger sauce (or other oil-free stir fry sauce) depending on preference
2 cups of broccoli florets
¼ cup of chopped jicama or water chestnuts sliced or chopped depending on your preference
2 scallions chopped
¼ cup fresh basil or Thai basil chopped (optional)
1-2 tbsp of ground dry roasted nuts (cashews, almonds, etc.) sprinkled on top (optional)

1. In a large, hot, non-stick skillet add onions and water and sauté for a couple of minutes.
2. Then add the garlic and ginger and continue to sauté until golden.
3. Add more water as necessary (1 tbsp at a time, just enough to keep from burning).
4. Then add shredded carrots, mushrooms, and eggplant and continue to water sauté (adding water as needed) until soft.
5. Then add the soy ginger sauce, broccoli, and scallions and cover and cook until broccoli is desired tenderness.
6. Then add basil, stir and serve over steamed brown rice.

NOTE: if you like, you could use a peanut sauce instead of the soy ginger sauce (see peanut sauce recipe)

✸

Tomato Basil Pizza

1 Nature's Highlights oil-free pizza crust (or another crust of your choice)
2 medium tomatoes chopped
1 small red onion chopped
2 cloves garlic chopped
1 tbsp dried basil (can substitute 3 tbsp of fresh basil but use towards the end of preparation)
1 box mushrooms chopped, cooked
Other ingredients optional (pineapple, peppers, broccoli, etc.)
1-2 cups oil-free tomato sauce (optional)
1-2 tbsp Vegan Parma or nutritional yeast (enough to sprinkle across entire pizza) OR spread with cashew sauce (see cashew sauce in Mac N 'Cheese' recipe)
½ cup fresh chopped arugula (optional)

1. Heat up Nature's Highlights oil-free pizza crust (or another crust of your choice) per instructions on box.
2. In a hot pan sauté (with oil-free liquid such as water, juice, broth, etc.) tomatoes, onions, garlic, and basil until soft.
3. Then add mushrooms and cook until liquid is reduced.
4. Add other vegetables if desired.
5. Spread oil-free tomato sauce on pizza crust if desired.
6. Then place sautéed vegetables on the crust (with or without sauce).
7. Sprinkle Vegan Parma "cheese" or nutritional yeast on top and bake in oven per directions on box of crust or until thoroughly heated (note vegetables and crust should be lightly cooked already).
8. Then can sprinkle arugula on top to enhance with a nice peppery flavor.

An alternative to this is: (thank you Ellen Neufeld)
Added after cashew sauce is on pizza crust:
1. Add black beans, onions, bell peppers and avocado with some salsa to make a Mexican style pizza OR
2. Use fresh heirloom tomatoes (when available) with fresh basil leaves to make a more traditional pizza.

Desserts

Carrot Cake
(thank you Shoshana Pulde)

3 cups shredded carrots
¾ cups brown sugar
1 cup self-rising flour OR (1 cup flour, ½ tsp salt, 2 tsp baking powder, ½ tsp baking soda)
1 cup almond meal/flour
2 tsp cinnamon
½ cup orange juice
3 cups applesauce
1 cup golden raisins
1 cup chopped pecans (or walnuts)
3-4 oz can of unsweetened chopped pineapple

1. Preheat oven to 350 degrees.
2. Mix together (by hand) all the dry ingredients.
3. Mix raisins and nuts into dry ingredients to coat and separate
4. Add carrots, apple sauce, pineapple, and orange juice
5. Put the batter into a non-stick or silicon cake pan.
6. Bake for 45 minutes or until knife comes out clean when inserted in center.

Chocolate Balls
(thank you Shoshana Pulde)

This recipe is for about 12 balls.
5½ ounces of cocoa (Wonderslim fat free)
1 cup orange juice
1 cup brown sugar or 10-12 pitted dates
1 cup chopped pecans
1 cup raisins
2 tbsp vanilla or almond extract
2 cups almond meal/flour

If using sugar: Mix all ingredients together. Let sit for half an hour. Form balls and refrigerate.

If using dates: Put dates in a food processer to create a paste. Mix paste with the rest of the ingredients and let sit for half an hour. Form balls and refrigerate.

✳

Cupcakes with Peanut Butter Frosting
(thank you Rachel Lederman)

<u>Cupcakes</u>:
1 box chocolate cake mix (Whole Foods Brand without artificial ingredients)
1 15 oz can pumpkin
2 tbsp vanilla extract
soy/rice/oat milk according to the recipe (may not be necessary if you mix the ingredients well enough)

1. Mix ingredients together.
2. Bake according to the directions on the cake box.
3. After the cupcakes finish baking, let them cool.

<u>Peanut Butter Frosting</u>:
Heat 3 tbsp peanut butter and dilute with a ¼ cup of water
Add agave nectar (a few squeezes) or maple syrup to taste

1. Mix ingredients.
2. Frost cupcakes.
3. Enjoy.

Note: May be refrigerated if desired.

Appendix J: Testimonials

In April of 2009, Exsalus Health & Wellness Center gave me the opportunity to change my life, and boy has it! At the time, I was a type II diabetic taking nine pills and two shots daily. The doctors at Exsalus explained to me that I had the power to change this, and that they would give me the tools and the knowledge to be able to stop my medications and learn a new way of eating. I have been under their care for five months now and have lost approx 40 pounds and no longer need my medication. This life-changing experience has taught me a much better way to fuel my body, and by following the Exsalus Program I have also begun healing myself. By doing this and also incorporating an exercise program into my routine, I'm living a completely new Life! No pills, no shots, 40 pounds lighter, pant size 36-38 down to 32-33, and I feel better now than I have felt in years. Matt and Alona, I hope you understand how much you have changed my life. I am 54 years old and have never been in better health. THANK YOU SO MUCH! IT REALLY WORKED!

—Joey Aucoin, FL

"I have struggled with my weight my entire life. My first memory of being put on a diet was in the fifth grade, and that began a seemingly endless spiral of different diets, eating plans and fitness routines, all of which promised results, none of which delivered over the long haul. Despite following a vegetarian diet for nearly 10 years now, and being vegan for more than 5 of them, my weight continued to be a problem. Some months ago, I decided to get serious and look into something life-changing; something that would change me on a fundamental level.

Enter Exsalus Health & Wellness Center. Alona and Matt examined every aspect of my lifestyle, from what I ate and my level of physical activity down to sunlight exposure, general mood and sleep habits, and, after a good deal of discussion and consideration, were able to put together a program that fit me perfectly. Now, at age 42, I have lost over 30 pounds with next to no effort (and I'm still dropping weight), I eat as much food as I want, I'm physically active, and have seen a major turnaround in my overall health and sense of well-being. I wouldn't hesitate to suggest their program to anyone who wants to experience optimal health and wellness, as they've changed my life in the most profound way imaginable."

—William Faith, CA

"When I first met Dr. Lederman and Dr. Pulde, I had already lost about 44 pounds in about a year and a half. I was battling with type 2 diabetes, asthma, pains in my hips and joints, and had hit a weight loss plateau and was feeling pretty lousy in general. Frustrated with the constant sugar spikes and being on medicine that I really didn't want to take, I was ready to make a change to feel better, get healthy and lose the rest of the weight...I knew it was time for a change so I committed to the [Exsalus] program for 3 months.

...I finished the 3-month commitment I agreed to and felt so great that I have continued on the program. I have been on the program 4 months now and have lost 23 pounds, I am off of the diabetes medicine and the daily asthma medicine, and am pretty much asthma-free at this point. I have more energy and my blood sugar is pretty much under control, and I am looking forward to being diabetes-free in the near future.

This program does require commitment and time; however, how much time have I spent feeling sick and tired in comparison? I highly recommend this program for anyone who has any type of health issue, and also for anyone that just wants to feel better overall..."
—Leslie McKenna, CA

"...How many times are you frustrated because doctors simply don't care until you give them boatloads of money to see them for 2 minutes?? The doctors at Exsalus actually sat down with me for HOURS to discuss lifestyle changes that can prevent diseases and perfect my health...Also their answers make sense. They actively research about pretty much everything to ensure that their information is unbiased and benefits YOU, rather than some pharmaceutical company.

They are some of the very few honest, knowledgeable doctors you could ever find in Southern California. Many people fly out here to see them..."
—Yoon Kyung Park, CA

"I spent my younger years working at a pharmacy counter. Taking care of numerous customers over 65, on copious amounts of prescriptions, had a deep impact on my life - and I swore to myself I would find a different way to live. Now, as I find myself in my 40's waking up with aches and pains, having trouble sleeping due to stress and feeling an overall decline in my energy, I felt it was time to take my health seriously. Since going to Exsalus and learning so many truths behind nutrition from Alona and Matt, I know I am on the right path I had always wished for. Since making simple changes to my eating and cooking habits, I have felt a profound change within my approach to food as well as my health. I am gradually going down to ideal weight while eating healthy, delicious food all day, and I feel so much stronger and happier."

—Monica Richards, CA

"I was referred to Dr. Lederman and Dr. Pulde at Exsalus Health and Wellness Center (www.exsalus.com) through a well known physician, author, and nutritional specialist on the East Coast. I was searching for an intelligent, informed approach to getting and staying healthy. I am very selective about obtaining medical advice, because there is so much noise in the medical system today...alternative conflicting opinions, alternative conflicting diet programs, and physicians who are rushed to provide time for their patients.

What I found at Exsalus are deeply caring physicians who are dedicated to understanding the truth about obtaining optimum health and willing to take whatever time it takes with their patients to explain what needs to get done, answer all questions, and provide ongoing support. I am also impressed with the network of providers linked to Exsalus who can provide comprehensive advice, including cooking classes and therapies to help those trying to make life-altering changes for superior health.

Drs. Matt Lederman and Alona Pulde provide a comprehensive system of advice, support and medical care. For those with a desire to maximize their overall health and well-being, I cannot make any higher recommendation than seeking out their advice."

—Richard Taggart, CA

Appendix K: Carnivores versus Herbivores

For years, theorists have disagreed as to whether humans are herbivores, carnivores, or omnivores.[169,170] Although widely considered omnivores because of our ability to metabolize both animal and plant foods, many argue that a closer look at our anatomy and physiology will tell a different story. The following are some of the observations that were made which we found interesting. You can take it or leave it...just make sure to read it before you decide.

Oral Cavity/Teeth:
Carnivores and omnivores have large, wide mouths to help them tear into and firmly grasp their prey. Their jaws are built like simple hinges moving up and down primarily. This prevents them from properly chewing food, but they do not need to chew as they swallow food whole. They have piercing incisors, long and sharp canines, and molars with blade like edges, all to aid them in ripping through flesh.

In comparison, herbivores and humans have smaller mouths with jaws that move up and down as well as forward and from side to side, which allows for crushing and grinding. To further assist with chewing, they have broad flat incisors, small blunt canines, and square flat molars.

Saliva:
Because carnivores and omnivores generally swallow their food whole, they do not require digestive enzymes in their saliva. Herbivores and humans, on the other hand, rely on digestive enzymes in saliva to mix with and help further break down our pre-chewed food.

Nails/Claws:
Carnivores and omnivores have claws to help them capture their prey. Because herbivores and humans do not generally capture prey with their hands, they do not need claws. Instead, they have flat nails or rounded hooves.

Gastro-Intestinal Tract:
Carnivores and omnivores have large stomachs, which help them store their less frequently eaten meals. Their intestinal tracts, however, are short (about 3-6 times their body length), allowing them to pass their meat through before it rots. Herbivores and humans have

smaller stomachs and much longer intestinal tracts (10-12 times their body length). These long intestines allow enough time for plant foods to be broken down, digested, and absorbed.

Because their intestines are short and smooth, carnivores and omnivores do not require fiber in their diets. Herbivores and humans, on the other hand, need fiber to help prevent rotting of food by pushing it through their longer digestive tracts.

Finally, carnivores and omnivores have very acidic stomach contents (pH 1-2) to help them not only break down food but also to kill any bacteria commonly found on rotting meat. Herbivores and humans who do not generally consume inadequately chewed meat and bones, on the other hand, have significantly less acidic stomach contents (ph 4-5).

Cholesterol:
Carnivores are able to remove cholesterol much better than humans. The health of carnivores and omnivores is not harmed by a high-cholesterol diet. Unfortunately, humans do not share the same fate, and high cholesterol in our diets often leads to clogging of the arteries and heart disease.

Again, this is included to offer you one more thing to ponder...or not. Our take-home message here comes from William Shakespeare's famous quote, "What's in a name? That which we call a rose by any other name would smell as sweet." In essence, who cares what we are called or labeled? What is important to remember is that although humans may be able to metabolize and survive on a meat-based diet (a survival advantage for times of famine), our goal is not just to survive but to thrive, and that we do best on a plant-based diet.

Appendix L: Recommended Reading

Breaking the Food Seduction: The Hidden Reasons Behind Food Cravings---And 7 Steps to End Them Naturally, by Neal Barnard, MD, St. Martin's Griffin 2004.

The China Study: The Most Comprehensive Study of Nutrition Ever Conducted and the Startling Implications for Diet, Weight Loss and Long-term Health, by T. Colin Campbell, PhD and Thomas M. Campbell II, Benbella Books 2006.

Dr. McDougall's Digestive Tune-Up, by John A. McDougall, MD, Healthy Living Publications, 2006.

Dr. Neal Barnard's Program for Reversing Diabetes: The Scientifically Proven System for Reversing Diabetes without Drugs, by Neal Barnard, MD, Rodale Books 2008.

eCornell Certificate in Plant Based Nutrition, http://www.tcolincampbell.org/courses-resources/courses/

The Easy Way to Stop Smoking, Allen Carr, Sterling 2005.

The Engine 2 Diet: The Texas Firefighter's 28-Day Save-Your-Life Plan that Lowers Cholesterol and Burns Away the Pounds, Rip Esselstyn, Wellness Central 2009.

The McDougall Health-Supporting Cookbook: Volume Two, by Mary McDougall, New Win Publishing 1986.

The McDougall Plan, by John A. McDougall, MD, Plume, 1995.

The McDougall Program: 12 Days to Dynamic Health, by John A. and Mary McDougall, MD, Plume, 1991.

The McDougall Program for a Healthy Heart: A Life-Saving Approach to Preventing and Treating Heart Disease, by John A. McDougall, MD, Plume 1998.

The McDougall Program for Maximum Weight Loss, by John A. McDougall, MD, Plume 1995.

The McDougall Program for Women, by John A. McDougall, MD, Plume 2000.

The McDougall Quick and Easy Cookbook: Over 300 Delicious Low-Fat Recipes You Can Prepare in Fifteen Minutes or Less, by John A. and Mary McDougall, MD, Plume 1999.

McDougall's Medicine: A Challenging Second Opinion, by John A. McDougall, MD, Smithmark Pub 1988.

The New McDougall Cookbook: 300 Delicious Ultra-Low-Fat Recipes, by John A. and Mary McDougall, MD, Plume 1997.

Overdosed America: The Broken Promise of American Medicine, John Abramson, MD, Harper Perennial 2008.

The Pleasure Trap, by Douglas J. Lisle, Ph.D. and Alan Goldhamer, D.C., Book Publishing Co. 2006.

Prevent and Reverse Heart Disease: The Revolutionary, Scientifically Proven, Nutrition-Based Cure, by Caldwell B. Esselstyn, Jr., MD, Avery Trade 2008.

The RAVE Diet & Lifestyle, by Mike Anderson, RaveDiet.com 2009.

Selling Sickness: How the World's Biggest Pharmaceutical Companies Are Turning Us All into Patients, by Ray Moynihan and Alan Cassels, Nation Books 2005.

Should I Be Tested for Cancer?: Maybe Not and Here's Why, by H. Gilbert Welch, MD, MPH, University of California Press 2006.

References

[1] Harvey and Marilyn Diamond, *Fit For Life* (New York: Warner Books,1985).

[2] Dr. David Katz, director of Yale prevention research center, April 2005.

[3] W.H.O. 1996; Japan Ministry of Health and Welfare 2004; U.S. Department of Health and Human Services/CDC 2005.

[4] www.cdc.gov/nchs/fastats/overwt.htm (accessed 9/14/09)

[5] Wang, Toufa, et al. Will all Americans become overweight or obese? Estimating the progression and cost of the U.S. obesity epidemic. Obesity (2008)16,2323-30.

[6] www.cdc.gov/nchs/fastats/overwt.htm (accessed 9/14/09)

[7] Wise, RA Dopamine and reward: the anhedonia hypothesis 30 years on. Neurotox Res. 2008 Oct;14(2-3):169-83.

[8] Lisle DJ, Goldhamer A *The Pleasure Trap:Mastering the Hidden Force That Undermines Health and Happiness* (Healthy Living Publications, 2006).

[9] Ibid

[10] Dr. David Katz, director of Yale prevention research center, April 2005.

[11] OECD Life Expectancy in OECD countries in 2003.

[12] WHO Issues New Healthy Life Expectancy Rankings, Press Release WHO, Released in Washington, D.C. and Geneva, Switzerland, 4 June 2000.

[13] OECD Health Data 2006 How Does the United States Compare.

[14] www.cdc.gov/nchs/fastats/overwt.htm (accessed 9/14/09)

[15] Barbara Starfield, MD, MPH, Is U.S. Health Really the Best in the World? JAMA, Volume 284, No. 4, July 26, 2000.

[16] Bates DW, Cullen DJ, Laird N, et al. Incidence of adverse drug events and potential adverse drug events. Implications for prevention. ADE Prevention Study Group. JAMA. 1995 Jul 5;274(1):29-34.

[17] Abramson J, MD Overdosed America (Harper Perennial, 2005).

[18] Anne Kavangh, PhD; Heather Mitchell, MD; Graham G Giles, PhD Hormone replacement therapy and accuracy of mammographic screening The Lancet Vol 355, Issue 9200 January 22, 2000, pages 270-274.

[19] Lowe GD. Hormone replacement therapy and cardiovascular disease: increased risks of venous thromboembolism and stroke, and no protection from coronary heart disease. J Intern Med. 2004 Nov;256(5):361-74.

[20] Chi-Ling Chen, PhD; Noel S. Weiss, MD, DrPH; Polly Newcomb, PhD; William Barlow, PhD; Emily White, PhD Hormone Replacement

Therapy in Relation to Breast Cancer JAMA, 2002;Vol 287, No. 6, Feb 2002:734-741.

[21] Brody, Howard MD, PhD The Company We Keep: Why Physician's Should Refuse to See Pharmaceutical Representatives. Annals of Family Medicine, Vol 3, No. 1, January/February 2005.

[22] Choudhry NK, Stelfox HT, Detsky AS. Relationships between authors of clinical practice guidelines and the pharmaceutical industry. JAMA 2002;287:612-7

[23] http://www.nhlbi.nih.gov/guidelines/groups.htm#disclosure (accessed 9/14/09)

[24] Blumenthal, David. Academic-industrial relationships in the life sciences. NEJM. December 18, 2003, number 25, Volume 349:2452-2459 and Agence France-Presse (AFP) June 2006; www.naturalnews.com/019981.html

[25] Bodil Als-Nielsen, MD; Wendong Chen, MD; Christian Gluud, MD, DMSc; Lise L. Kjaergard, MD Association of Funding and Conclusions in Randomized Drug Trials: A Reflection of Treatment Effect or Adverse Events? JAMA 2003; 290;921-928.

[26] Blumenthal, David. Academic-industrial relationships in the life sciences. NEJM. December 18, 2003, number 25, Volume 349:2452-2459.

[27] Wymer, Walter. A Macromarketing Analysis of Prescription Drugs in the US. Journal of Research for Consumers. Issue: 14, 2008. Quote on pg 6

[28] Constitution of the World Health Organization

[29] Hansson, Lennart. Antihypertensive Treatment: Does the J-curve Exist? Cardiovascular Drugs and Therapy 2000; 14:367-372.

[30] A compilation from the following sites: U.S. Bureau of Labor Statistics; http://ehealthplan.kp.org/ApplyOnline/ iQGetAgeGender.do;www.metlife.com/ WPSAssets/41453139101127828650V1F2005%20NH%20and%20HC%20Market %20Survey.pdf;http://www.usatoday.com/news/health/2006-05-01-gastric band_x.htm;http://myhealth.ucsd.edu/healthnews/ HealthNewsFeature/ hnf053104.htm;http://missourifamilies.org/quick/healthqa/ healthqa31.htm;http://yourtotalhealth.ivillage.com/cost-colonoscopy.html)

[31] Gerhauser, Clarissa. Cancer chemopreventative potential of apples, apple juice, and apple components. Planta Med 2008;74:1608-1624.

[32] He, Xiangjiu, et al. Phytochemicals of apple peels: isolation, structure, elucidation, and their antiproliferative and antioxidant activities. J Agric Food Chem, Vol. 56, No 21, 2008, pp. 9905-10.

[33] Park, H, et al. Genistein inhibits differentiation of primary human adipocytes. The Journal of Nutritional Biochemistry. Volume 20, issue 2, pp. 140-8, February 2009.

[34] Idea inspired by Lisle, DJ lecturing at the McDougall 10-day Program, January 2008.

[35] Lappe, Frances Moore Diet for a Small Planet, 10th Anniversary Ed.; 1982; p. 162.

[36] Rose, W.C., (1957) The Amino acid requirements of adult man. Nutr abstr. revs. 27: 631-647.

[37] Johnson, Julius and Haines, Williams. Role of Amino Acids in Human Nutrition. Journal of the Federation of American Societies for Experimental Biology. Volume 6, March 1992, pp. 2361-2.

[38] Ibid.

[39] Protein and amino acid requirements in human nutrition. Report of a Joint WHO/FAQ/UNU Expert Consultation. Technical Report Series, No 935. World Health Organization

[40] J Pennington. Bowes and Church's Food Values of Portions Commonly Used. 17th Ed. Lippincott. Philadelphia-New York. 1998.

[41] U.S. Department of Health and Human Services, National Institute of Health, The Kidneys and How They Work, NIH Publication No. 09–3195 February 2009.

[42] AJCN. A high ratio of dietary animal to vegetable protein increases the rate of bone loss and the risk of fracture in postmenopausal women. Vol. 73, No. 1, 118-122, January 2001.

[43] Key TJ. Body mass index, serum sex hormones, and breast cancer risk in postmenopausal women. J Natl Cancer Inst. 2003 Aug 20;95(16):1218-26.

[44] Peterson, Kitt, et al. Impaired Mitochondrial Activity in the Insulin-Resistant Offspring of Patients with Type 2 Diabetes. N Engl J Med 2004;350:664-71.

[45] Hu, Jinfu. Meat and Fish consumption and cancer in Canada. Nutrition and cancer, 60(3),313-24.

[46] Sinha, et al. Meat Intake and Mortality: A Prospective Study of Over Half a Million People. Archives of Internal Medicine, 2009; 169 (6): 562.

[47] Stripp C, Overvad K, Christensen J, Thomsen BL, Olsen A, Moller S, Tjonneland A. Fish intake is positively associated with breast cancer incidence rate. J Nutr. 2003 Nov;133(11):3664-9.

[48] EPA PCB's Update: Impact on Fish Advisories, Sept 1999.

[49] Guallar, et al. Mercury, fish oils, and the risk of myocardial infarction. NEJM 2002, 11/28; 347(22):1747-54.

[50] Jacobson, et al. Intellectual impairment in children exposed to polychlorinated biphenyls in utero. NEJM. Volume 335:783-789. 9/12/1996. Number 11 pp.783-9

[51] Tryphonas, Helen. The impact of PCBs and Dioxins on Children's Health: Immunological Considerations. Canadian Journal of Public Health. Volume 89, supplements 1 pp S49-52.

[52] Schantz, et al. Effects of PCB exposure on neuropsychological function in children. Environmental Health Perspectives. Vol . 111, 2003.

[53] Guallar, et al. Mercury, fish oils, and the risk of myocardial infarction. NEJM 2002, 11/28; 347(22):1747-54.

[54] Schecter, Arnold, et al. Intake of dioxins and related compounds from food in the U.S. population. Journal of Toxicology and Environmental Health, Part A, 63:1–18, 2001.

[55] EPA, Polychlorinated Biphenyls (PCBs) Update: Impact on Fish Advisories, Sept 1999

[56] Ibid

[57] Public Health Implications of Exposure to Polychlorinated Biphenyls (PCBs) – A report by the Agency for Toxic Substances and Disease Registry (ATSDR) and the U.S. Environmental Protection Agency (EPA). You can view the assessment in full at http://www.atsdr.cdc.gov /DT/pcb007.html (accessed 9/14/09)

[58] Niederau, C, et al. Epidemiology, clinical spectrum and prognosis of hemochromatosis. Adv Exp Med Biol 1994; 356:293-302.

[59] Wurapa, et al. Primary iron overload in African Americans. Am J Med. 1996 Jul; 101(1):9-18.

[60] Niederau, C, et al. Epidemiology, clinical spectrum, and prognosis of hemochromatosis. Adv Exp Med Biol 1994;356:293.

[61] Zacharski, L, et al. Decreased cancer risk after iron reduction in patients with peripheral arterial disease: results from a randomized trial. J Natl Cancer Inst 2008;100:996-1002.

[62] Adlercreutz H. Phyto-estrogens and cancer. Lancet Oncol. 2002 Jun;3(6):364-73.

[63] Iwasaki, Motoki, et al. Plasma isoflavone level and subsequent risk of breast cancer among Japanese women: a nested case-control study from the Japan public health center-based prospective study group. Journal of Clinical Oncology. Volume 26, number 10, April 1, 2008, 1677-83.

[64] Fink, Brian, et al. Dietary Flavonoid Intake and Breast Cancer Survival among Women on Long Island. Cancer Epidemio Biomarkers Prev 2007:16(11). November 2007, pp. 2285-92.

[65] Jenkins D. Effects of high- and low-isoflavone soy foods on blood lipids, oxidized LDL, homocysteine, and blood pressure in hyperlipidemic men and women. Am J Clin Nutr. 2002 Aug;76(2):365-72.

[66] Anderson JW, Johnstone BM, Cook-Newell ME Meta-analysis of the effects of soy protein intake on serum lipids. N Engl J Med. 1995 Aug 3;333(5):276-82.

[67] American Heart Association (AHA) Comments to FDA on Soy Protein and Coronary Heart Disease Health Claim, May 1, 2008.

[68] Yellayi S. The phytoestrogen genistein induces thymic and immune changes: a human health concern? Proc Natl Acad Sci USA. 2002 May 28:99(11):7616-21.

[69] Jenkins DJ, Kendall CW, Connelly PW, Jackson CJ, Parker T, Faulkner D, Vidgen E. Effects of high- and low- isoflavone (phytoestrogen) soy foods on inflammatory biomarkers and proinflammatory cytokines in middle-aged men and women. Metabolism. 2002 Jul;51(7):919-24.

[70] Doerge DR, Sheehan DM. Goitrogenic and estrogenic activity of soy isolfavones. Environ Health Perspect. 2002 Jun;110 Suppl 3:349-53.

[71] Horn-Ross PL, Hoggatt KJ, Lee MM. "Phytoestrogens and thyroid cancer risk: the San Francisco bay Area thyroid cancer study." Cancer Epidemiol Biomarkers Prev. 2002 Jan;11(1):43-9.

[72] Arjmandi BH, Khalil DA, Smith BJ, Lucas EA, Juma S, Payton ME, Wild RA. Soy protein has a greater effect on bone in postmenopausal women not on hormone replacement therapy, as evidenced by reducing bone resorption and urinary calcium excretion. J Clin Endocrinol Metab. 2003 Mar;88(3):1048-54.

[73] Khalil DA, Lucas EA, Juma S, Smith BJ, Payton ME, Arjmadi BH "Soy Protein Supplementation Increases Serum Insulin-Like Growth Factor-1 in Young and Old Men but Does Not Affect Markers of Bone Metabolism. J. Nutr. 132:2605-2608, September 2002.

[74] Nagata, C, et al. Decreased Serum Total Cholesterol Concentration Is Associated with High Intake of Soy Products in Japanese Men and Women. Journal of Nutrition (1998) 128:209-213.

[75] Novick, Jeff. Putting Soy Consumption in Perspective, Feb 2008 18:56.

[76] Paterson CR. Calcium requirements in man: a critical review. Postgrad Med J. 1978 Apr;54(630):244-8.

[77] Ibid

[78] FAO/WHO Expert Group. Calcium Requirements. Rome: Food and Agriculture Organziation 1962.

[79] Lanou AJ, Berkow SE, Barnard ND. Calcium, dairy products, and bone health in children and young adults: a reevaluation of the evidence. Pediatrics. 2005 Mar;115(3):736-43.

[80] Winzenberg T, Shaw K, Fryer J, Jones G. Effects of calcium supplementation on bone density in healthy children: meta-analysis of randomized controlled trials. BMJ. 2006 Oct 14;333(7572):775.

[81] Lanou AJ. Bone health in children. *BMJ.* 2006 Oct 14;333(7572):763-4.

[82] Cumming RG, Klineberg RJ Case-Control Study of Risk Factors for Hip Fractures in the Elderly. American Journal of Epidemiology Vol. 139, No. 5:493-503.

[83] Feskanich, Diane, et al. Milk, dietary Calcium, and Bone Fractures in Women: A 12-Year Prospective Study. American Journal of Public Health, June 1997, Vol 87, No. 6, pp. 992-7.

[84] Hegsted, D. M. Calcium and Osteoporosis. J. Nutr. 116. 2316-2319, 1986.

[85] Kolata G How Important is dietary calcium in preventing osteoporosis? Science Aug 1986;Vol 233, no. 4763;519-520.

[86] Allen LH, Oddoye EA, Margen S Protein-induced hypercalciuria: a longer term study. American Journal of Clinical Nutrition 1979 Vol 32(4), 741-749.

[87] MJ McKenna, et al. Safety and efficacy of increasing wintertime vitamin D and calcium intake by milk fortification. Q J Med 1995; 88: 895-898.

[88] Holick, MF Environmental factors that influence the cutaneous production of vitamin D. Am J Clin Nutr. 1995 Mar;61(3Suppl):638S-645S.

[89] Barr, Susan Increased Dairy Product or Calcium Intake: Is Body Weight or Composition Affected in Humans? J. Nutr. 133:245S-248S, January 2003.

[90] Ibid

[91] Radak, T; Lanou A; Barnard N The Dairy and Weight Loss Hypothesis: An Evaluation of the Evidence. Nutr Rev. 2008 May;66(5):272-9.

[92] Iacono, Giuseppe, et al. Intolerance of cow's milk and chronic constipation in children. NEJM, volume 339: number 16, October 15, 1998, pp 1100-04.

[93] Saukkonen T, etal Significance of cow's milk protein antibodies as risk factor for childhood IDDM: interactions with dietary cow's milk intake and HLA-DQB1 genotype. Childhood Diabetes in Finland Study Group. Diabetologia. 1998 Jan;41(1):72-8.

[94] Fava D. etal Relationship between dairy product consumption and incidence of IDDM in childhood in Italy. Diabetes Care. 1994 Dec;17(12):1488-90.

[95] Dahl-Jorgensen K. etal Relationship between cows' milk consumption and incidence of IDDM in childhood. Diabetes Care. 1991 Nov;14(11):1081-3.

[96] Heaney, RP, et al. Dietary changes favorably affect bone remodeling in older adults. J Am Diet Assoc. 2002 Nov;102(11):1672-4.

[97] Moschos SJ, Mantzoros CS. The role of IGF system in cancer: from basic to clinical studies and clinical applications. Oncology. 2002;63(4):317-32.

[98] Van der Pols, JC, etal Childhood dairy intake and adult cancer risk: 65-y follow-up of the Boyd Orr cohort. Am J Clin Nutr. 2007 Dec;86(6):1722-9.

[99] Hankinson, S. E., et al. Circulating concentrations of insulin-like growth factor-I and risk of breast cancer. The Lancet, Vol. 351, May 9, 1998, pp. 1393-96.

[100] Chan JM, Stampfer MJ, Ma J, Gann PH, Gaziano JM, Giovannucci E. Dairy products, calcium, and prostate cancer risk in the Physicians' Health Study. Am J Clin Nutr 2001;74:549-54.

[101] Pescovitz, Ora Hirsch, Eugster Erica A. Pediatric Endocrinology: Mechanisms and Management, Lippincott Williams & Wilkins, 2004

[102] Hartmann S, Lacorn M, Steinhart H. Natural occurrence of steroid hormones in food. Food Chem 1998; 62: 7-20.

[103] Schecter, A Intake of Dioxins and Related Compounds From Food in the U.S. Population. Journal of Toxicology and Environmental Health, Part A, 63:1-18, 2001.

[104] Gonda M. Bovine immunodeficiency virus. AIDS. 1992 Aug; 6(8):759-76.

[105] "You Can't Tell By Looking," Hoard's Dairyman (National Dairy Farm Magazine), Volume 147, Number 4, Feb 25, 2002.

[106] Gertrude Case Buehring, Sean M. Philpott, K. Yeon Choi. AIDS Research and Human Retroviruses – Humans Have Antibodies Reactive with Bovine Leukemia Virus. December 1, 2003, 19(12): 1105-1113.

[107] Buehring GC, Choi KY, Jensen HM Bovine leukemia virus in human breast tissues. Breast Cancer Res 2001, 3(Suppl 1):A14.

[108] Cosivi, O, etal. Zoonotic Tuberculosis due to Mycobacterium bovis in Developing Countries, Emerging Infectious Diseases. Volume 4, Number 1 January-March 1998.

[109] Ibid.

[110] www.cdc.gov/mmwr: Surveillance Summaries June 01,1988/37(SS-2);25-31.

[111] Dalton, C. An Outbreak of Gastroenteritis and Fever due to Listeria. monocytogenes in Milk. NEJM Volume 336:100-106. Jan 9,1997.Number 2.

[112] Hennessy, T. A National Outbreak of Salmonella enteritidis Infections from Ice Cream. NEJM Vol 334:1281-1286, May 16,1996, Number 20.

[113] Ackers, ML An outbreak of Yersinia enterocolitica O:8 infections associated with pasteurized milk. J Infect Dis. 2000 May;181(5):1834-7.

[114] Yuan, Jean W., Jay, M.T., et al, Campylobacteriosis Outbreak Associated with Pasteurized Milk — California, May 2006, Epidemic Intelligence Service Conference 2007 (CDC), 2007 APR 16; page 62.

[115] Cumming, M, et al. Outbreak of Listeria monocytogenes Infections Associated With Pasteurized Milk From a Local Dairy— Massachusetts, 2007.JAMA. 2009;301(8):820-822.

[116] Meisel, Hans, et al. Opioid peptides encrypted in intact milk protein sequences. British Journal of Nutrition (2000),84,Suppl.1,S27-S31.

[117] Panksepp, J, et al. Casomorphins reduce separation distress in chicks. Peptides 1984;5:829-31

[118] Ginsberg, Henry N., etal Effects of Reducing Dietary Saturated Fatty Acids on Plasma Lipids and Lipoproteins in Healthy Subjects: The Delta Study, Protocol 1. Arteriosclerosis, Thrombosis & Vascular Biology. 18(3):441-449, March 1998.

[119] http://www.americanheart.org/presenter.jhtml?identifier=4582 (accessed 9/14/09)

[120] Letter Report on dietary reference intakes for Trans Fatty Acids, Food and Nutrition Board, Institute of Medicine. http://www.iom.edu/CMS/5410.aspx.

[121] Preventing Childhood Obesity: Health in the Balance 2005, Institute of Medicine

[122] Center for Disease Control: Overweight and Obesity Publications and Materials

[123] http://www.iom.edu/CMS/54133/54377.aspx) (accessed 9/14/09 "summary statement)

[124] Stripp C, Overvad K, Christensen J, Thomsen BL, Olsen A, Moller S, Tjonneland A. Fish intake is positively associated with breast cancer incidence rate. J Nutr. 2003 Nov;133(11):3664-9.

[125] Davis, Brenda, et al. Achieving Optimal Essential Fatty Acid Status in Vegetarians: Current Knowledge and Practical Implications. Am J Clin Nutr 2003; 78(suppl):640S-6S.

[126] Simopoulos, A.P. Human Requirement for N-3 Polynunsaturated Fatty Acids Poult Sci 2000 Jul; 79(7):961-70.

[127] Horrobin, David. Fatty acid metabolism in health and disease: the role of delta-6-desaturase. American Journal of Clinical Nutrition 1993;57(suppl):732S-7S.

[128] Simopoulos, AP. The importance of the ratio of omega-6/omega-3 essential fatty acids. Biomed Pharmacother. 2002 Oct;56(8):365-79.

[129] Jeff Novick, MS, RD, LD, LN speaking at the January 2008 McDougall 10-Day Program. "From Oil to Nuts: The Essential Facts on Fats!"

[130] Manach, Claudine, et al. Polyphenols: food sources and bioavailability. Am J Clin Nutr. 2004;79:727– 47.

[131] American Heart Association Nutrition and Cardiovascular Diseases – Statistics

[132] Jeff Novick, MS, RD, LD, LN speaking at the January 2008 McDougall 10-Day Program. "From Oil to Nuts: The Essential Facts on Fats!"

[133] Blankenhorn, David, et al. The influence of diet on the appearance of new lesions in human coronary arteries. JAMA, March 23/30. 1990, Vol 263. No. 12, pp 1646-52.

[134] Rudel, Lawrence, et al. Compared with dietary monounsaturated and saturated fat, polyunsaturated fat protects African Green Monkeys from coronary artery atherosclerosis. Arteriosclerosis, Thrombosis, and vascular biology. 1995;15:2101-10.

[135] Vogel, Robert, et al. The postprandial effect of components of the Mediterranean diet on endothelial function. J Am Coll Cardiol 2000;36:1455-60.

[136] Swank, Roy. Multiple sclerosis: the lipid relationship. Am J Clin Nutr 1988;48:1387-93.

[137] Cox, C, et al. Effects of dietary coconut oil, butter and safflower oil on plasma lipids, lipoproteins and lathosterol levels. European Journal of clinical nutrition. (1998)52, 650-54.

[138] Kalustian, Peter. Pharmaceutical and cosmetic uses of palm and lauric products. Journal of the American Oil Chemists' Society. Volume 62, Number 2 / February, 1985. & www.jeffnovick.com

[139] Marks, Dawn, et al. Basic Medical Biochemistry: A Clinical Approach. Lippincott Williams & Wilkins, Baltimore, Maryland. 1996.

[140] Hammer, Roger, et al. Calorie-restricted low-fat diet and exercise in obese women. American Journal of Clinical Nutrition. 1989;49:77-85.

[141] Rose, W.C., (1957) The Amino acid requirements of adult man. Nutr abstr. revs. 27: 631-647.

[142] Westman, Eric, et al. Effect of 6-month adherence to a very low carbohydrate diet program. American Journal of Medicine. Volume 113, Issue 1 Pages 30-36 (July 2002.

[143] Wing RR. Cognitive effects of ketogenic weight-reducing diets. Int J Obes Relat Metab Disord. 1995 Nov;19(11):811-6.

[144] Saris, Wim. Sugars, energy metabolism, and body weight control. American Journal of Clinical Nutrition. 2003;78(suppl):850S-7S.

[145] Hellerstein, Marc. No common energy currency: de novo lipogenesis as the road less traveled. American Journal of Clinical Nutrition. 2001;74:707-8.

[146] Chu, NF, et al. Dietary and lifestyle factors in relation to plasma leptin concentrations among normal weight and overweight men. International Journal of Obesity (2001) 25, 106-14.

[147] Perry, George, et al. Diet and the evolution of human amylase gene copy number variation. Nat Genet. 2007 October;39(10):1256-60.

[148] Levine AS, Kotz CM, Gosnell BA. Sugars: hedonic aspects, neuroregulation, and energy balance. Am J Clin Nutr. 2003 Oct;78(4):834S-842S.

[149] Niederau, C, et al. Epidemiology, clinical spectrum, and prognosis of hemochromatosis. Adv Exp Med Biol 1994;356:293.

[150] Arterburn, Linda, et al. Bioequivalence of Docosahexaenoic acid from different algal oils in capsules and in a DHA-fortified food. Lipids (2007) 42:1011-24.

[151] Bolland, Mark, et al. Vascular events in healthy older women receiving calcium supplementation: randomized controlled trial. BMJ 2008; DOI:10.1136/ bmj. 39440.525752.BE

[152] Agus ZS, Morad M. Modulation of cardiac ion channels by magnesium. Annu Rev Physiol. 1991;53:299-307.

[153] Feskanich D; Singh V; Willett WC; Colditz GA Vitamin A intake and hip fractures among postmenopausal women JAMA 2002 Jan 2;287(1):47-54.

[154] Bjelakovic, Goran. Mortality in randomized trials of antioxidant supplements for primary and secondary prevention: systematic review and meta-analysis. JAMA. 2007;297(8):842-57.

[155] Acuna, Juan, et al. "The prevention of neural tube defects with folic acid." CDC report: Pan American Health Organization.

[156] Ibid

[157] Ibid

[158] Charles, Deborah, et al. Taking folate in pregnancy and risk of maternal breast cancer. BMJ 2004;329:1375–6.

[159] http://dietary-spplements.info.nih.gov/factsheets/folate.asp#h10 (accessed 9/14/09)

[160] Hicks, Penni, et al. Iron deficiency but not anemia upregulates iron absorption in breast fed Peruvian infants. J. Nutr. 136:2435-2438,2006.

[161] McCormick, Charles. Passive diffusion does not play a major role in the absorption of dietary calcium in normal adults. Journal of Nutrition. 2002. 132:3428-3430.

[162] Taking Vitamin Supplements To Prevent Cardiovascular Disease and Cancer: Recommendations from the U.S. Preventive Services Task Force. Annals of Internal Medicine 1 July 2003 | Volume 139 Issue 1 | Page I-76)

[163] Dusseldorp, Marijke, et al. Risk of persistent cobalamin deficiency in adolescents fed a macrobiotic diet in early life. Am J Clin Nutr 1999;69:664-71.

[164] Melamed, Michael, et al. 25-hydroxyvitamin D levels and the risk of mortality in the general population. Arch Intern Med. Vol 168(No. 15), Aug 11/25, 2008, pp. 1629-37.

[165] Autier, Philippe, et al. Vitamin D supplementation and total mortality. Arch Intern Med. 2007;167(16);1730-1737.

[166] Witham, Miles. More evidence is needed before general supplementation. BMJ, 2008; 336: 1451 (28 June).

[167] Nelemans, Patty, et al. Effect of Intermittent exposure to sunlight on melanoma risk among indoor workers and sun-sensitive individuals. Environmental Health Perspectives. 101:252-255, 1992.

[168] Kent ST, McClure LA, Crosson WI, Arnett DK, Wadley VG, Sathiakumar N "Effect of sunlight exposure on cognitive function among depressed and non-depressed participants: a REGARDS cross-sectional study." Environ Health. 2009 Jul 28;8:34.

[169] from: Cardiologist William C. Roberts editor in chief of The American Journal of Cardiology and medical director of the Baylor Heart and Vascular Institute (Deneen, Sally, "Body of evidence: were humans meant to eat meat?" The Environmental Magazine, Jan-Feb 2002)

[170] Mills, Milton R. MD The Comparative Anatomy of Eating.

Index

Notes

Notes